JUSTICE
for the
HEALTH *of It*
#HEALTHJUSTICE

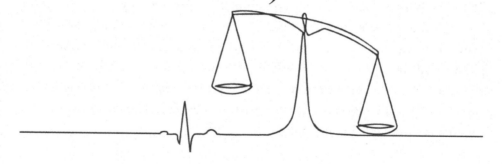

D1257378

DR. LATRICE D. SNODGRASS

Published by *Self Publish -N- 30 Days*

Printed in the United States of America
ISBN: 979-8-53273-287-2
1. Health Disparity 2. Informational 3. Racial Justice
Dr. LaTrice Snodgrass *JUSTice for the Health of It*

Disclaimer/Warning:
This book is intended for lecture and informative purposes only. This publication is designed to provide competent and reliable information regarding the subject matter covered. The author or publisher are not engaged in rendering legal or professional advice. Laws vary from state to state and if legal, financial, or other expert assistance is needed, the services of a professional should be sought. The author and publisher disclaim any liability that is incurred from the use or application of the contents of this book.

THIS BOOK IS DEDICATED TO:

The Gatekeepers
*Anyone that can influence equity through advocacy, policy and/or
granting access to services and resources.*
#DoTheRightThing

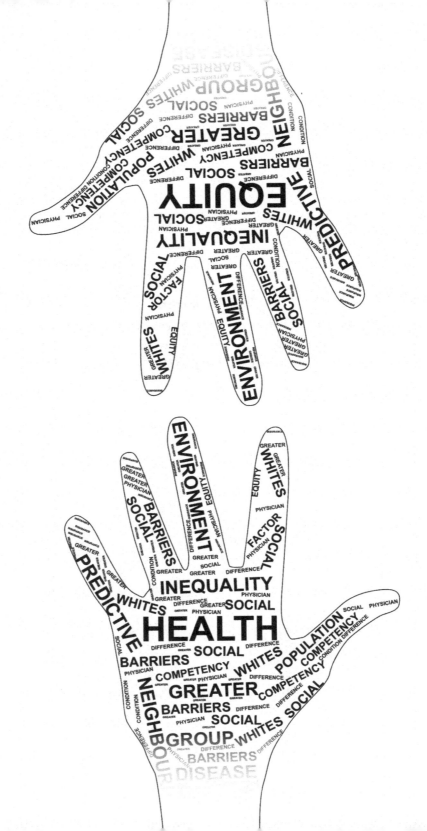

"Of all the forms of inequality, injustice in healthcare is the most shocking and inhumane."
— *Dr. Martin Luther King, Jr.*

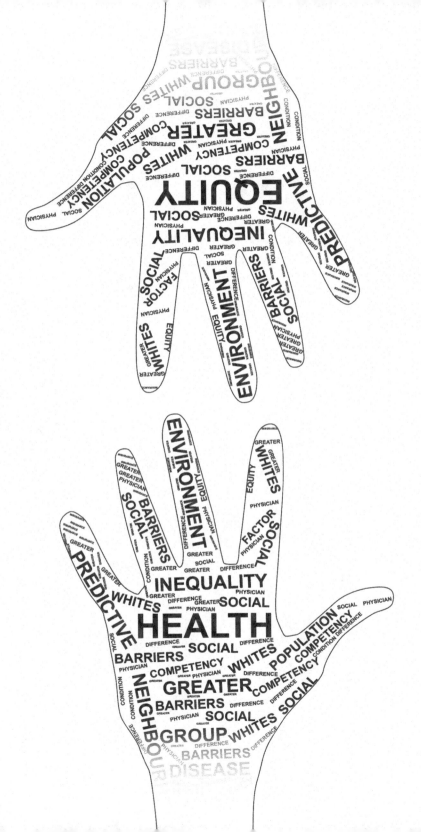

TABLE OF CONTENTS

Δ

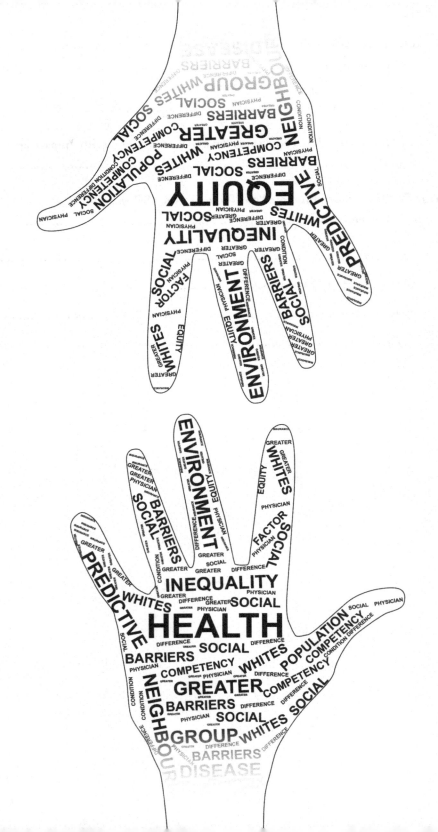

FOREWORD

Δ

I am an African American female physician who grew up in an inner city *neighborhood* in Cleveland, Ohio. I have experienced disparity in healthcare and the impact of social determinants of health firsthand.

I am grateful to have served as the medical director of a center for health equity, which afforded me the opportunity to address these issues in the community I served. The *neighborhood* is where I was fortunate to meet Dr. LaTrice Snodgrass.

When Dr. LaTrice walked into my office for a job interview, I was so happy to see someone with brown skin. Yes, I see color. Being an African American female physician in a male-dominated Caucasian profession, I get excited when I can work with people who understand my plight.

She would be the first African American manager for the health care organization that employed us both. Her intellect, compassion, and leadership skills are the best I have ever encountered. Dr. LaTrice has been a trailblazer since the day I met her.

She has implemented many services in the community and serves on boards as a voice and advocate for the underrepresented. Not only did she get the job of manager, but she also became a director and a COO. She is more than qualified to write this book. Dr. LaTrice has lived it, learned it, and practices it daily.

I have witnessed her journey and can attest to her truth. She is a thought leader, encouraging everyone she encounters to do better. It has been a pleasure seeing her prosper.

If you do not understand the social determinants of health, then you must read this book. Dr. Snodgrass dissects the meaning and its implications thoroughly. One of the most powerful statements (paraphrased) is: Your zip code can have a greater influence on your life expectancy than your genes.

Social determinants of health mean your surroundings determine or contribute to your health. It is amazing how many entities influence our health and the disparity that surrounds them: our home, the cleanliness of the air we breathe, the water we drink, the food we eat, our neighborhood and community, our access to doctors, and lack thereof, transportation, our job, our schools, and our level of activity.

She explores each of these entities with real-world examples that cultivate connection, empathy, and understanding.

This book is informational and actionable. If you are interested in learning what to do to fix the problem, keep reading. It is unique because of perspective, rawness, and realism. It tells you how to be better, how to do better, and what to do.

It covers politics and policies, medicine and spirituality, slavery and reparations, self-care and advocacy, health justice, personal stories, historical facts, thought-provoking questions, and heart-wrenching answers.

Sit back or forward, listen, and learn because she is going to take you to the *neighborhood*.

Teresa A. Myers, MD, MHSA
Primary Care Physician
Cleveland Clinic, Cleveland, Ohio

PREFACE

Δ

As a child, I grew up living in a housing project called Rainbow Acres on the northeast side of Canton, Ohio. That was my home from the time I began kindergarten until the summer entering my junior year of high school.

During those years, I was bussed to schools in affluent neighborhoods. I was the only Black person in most of my classes, and I quickly learned the impact of prejudice, racism, and soft bigotry, both implicit and explicit.

I was forced to learn to adapt, find balance, and co-exist in this space with very few individuals that shared my lived experience. I would, however, like to point out that I have no complaints, as it was the first stage of preparing me for the assignment God has over my life; fighting for *health justice*.

On April the 26th of 1992, at the age of nineteen, I gave birth to my son and spent the next three years raising him in subsidized housing while enrolled as a full-time college student with a part-time "work-study" job.

Like many other young mothers without access to essential financial security, I received Medicaid for health coverage, a monthly welfare check, and food stamps.

I can recall those days, as if they were yesterday, of being on Medicaid. I remember being treated like a "second-class" citizen, having medical clinicians and care team members talk *at* me and not *to* me, disregard my concerns and comments, not answer my questions directly, or just blow me off and not answer my questions at all.

I was made to feel ashamed and discounted because I was "in the system." I was pegged as *"one of those lazy, uneducated, non-compliant patients"* when no one really bothered to listen because, in their minds, I was *"that able-bodied person that was taking advantage of their tax money."*

I did not feel like an active participant in my own health and wellness journey. Although, at the time, I was unable to articulate "that," as I did not understand what "that" was.

I eventually got married, began working full-time, and put school on hold. Fortunately—although many years later—due to the dawn of online learning, I was afforded the opportunity to return to school and still work full-time.

Shortly thereafter, I was introduced to the field of healthcare and fell in love. My pathway was set because my passion resides in this space.

In 2005, I received my master's degree in Health Care Management, followed by a doctorate in Health Care Administration in 2015. Entering the healthcare arena as a professional staff member, I vowed that I would aim to make a difference for struggling people with marginalized backgrounds like my own.

Fast forward. Ever since that time, I have been laser-focused on ensuring that *all* people I encounter in my work in the healthcare field—regardless of their socioeconomic status, gender, or race—are treated with the most dignity and respect that I can afford them.

Perhaps it is because of my own personal struggles, but I am committed to aiding those fighting poverty and inequity.

First, as a medical assistant and then as an administrator, I have witnessed—over more than twenty years—how healthcare access, health outcomes, and health status of specific populations in the US are affected by social determinants of health (SDoH), leading to significant disparities.

Thus, I am focused on improving the SDoH that so frequently results in a lack of equitable care for marginalized populations. I have included all of this information about my own past so you can understand why I wrote this book, as well as why writing it was a "labor of love" for me.

My primary aims in creating this book were not to "place blame" but to draw attention and provide context that will foster thought-provoking dialogue about the issues contributing to healthcare inequities and promote an inclusive "call to action" to combat those imbalances.

It is my hope that after reading this book, you will better comprehend and gain compassion for how longstanding inequities based on "race" have fostered health disparities. My prayer is that you are better equipped to become a change agent and thereby promote equitable health care for all Americans.

Most of all, I am committed to moving the delivery of healthcare services from *transactional* to *transformational*. I hope that after reading this book, you will feel compelled to join me in this fight for *health justice*.

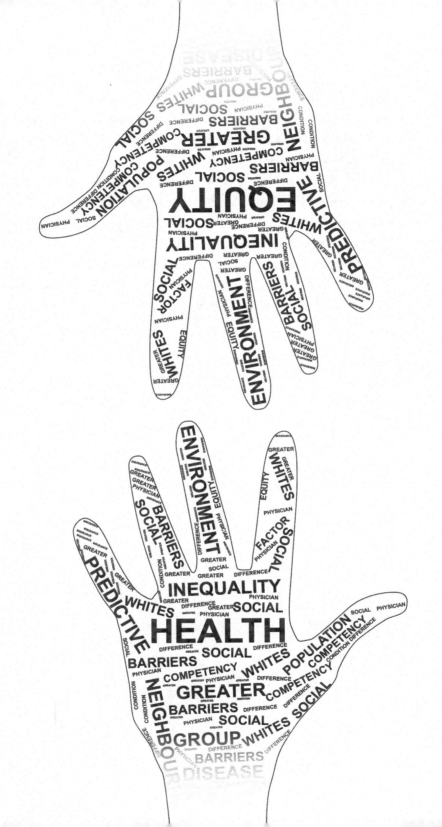

INTRODUCTION

Δ

In 1914, Booker T. Washington stated the following, in reference to the Black community: "Without health, and until we reduce the high death rate, it will be impossible for us to have permanent success in business, in property getting, in acquiring education, or to show other evidence of progress."

Over 100 years ago, he recognized the importance of population-impacting health inequity. This holds just as true in today's world.

Population health is a focus within the public health field concerned with the health experiences and outcomes of a group. It is an approach to health that aims to improve the condition of an entire population rather than considering the well-being (and obstacles to optimal health) of sole individuals.

Health imbalances are preventable variances in the burden of disease, injury, violence, healthcare access, treatment outcomes, and average life expectancy that are experienced by socially disadvantaged populations.

Worsened trends in all these population health measures are suffered by impoverished and marginalized populations throughout the United States.

Whether preventable health conditions fostered by lack of health care (and quality of that care), reduced utilization of care, or limited access to health insurance, socially *advantaged* populations fare better than socially *disadvantaged* populations in the US.

The two approaches that social justice advocates most commonly use to "level the playing field" and reduce health inequities are promoting equality and equity. While often used interchangeably, these terms are not the same.

From where I sit—in terms of healthcare provision—equality means that we treat everyone the same. It does not mean everyone is treated optimally. In contrast, equity means that we treat individuals based on what they need to thrive.

In *Healthy People 2020*[1], health inequities and health disparities are interchangeable terms that describe unbalanced health variations that adversely affect underserved populations.

Healthcare leaders must strive to implement processes, procedures, and practices to meet people at their place of need. It is only by understanding the underlying issues that cause gaps concurrent to inequity that the overall inequity can be addressed.

An individual's health outcomes are partially determined by how well one takes care of himself/herself and partially determined by other societal factors such as the potential for socioeconomic improvement.

Furthermore, some influences are conducive to better health regardless of social or socioeconomic status such as environmental factors inclusive of proximity to toxic hazards.

Indeed, living conditions, and the stressors that come with subpar living conditions, is an example of a health disparity category that has a notably adverse impact on underprivileged populations.

Healthcare leaders must strive to implement processes, procedures, and practices to meet people at their place of need.

Arlene Geronimus—a public health researcher in Michigan—coined the term *weathering*. This is the word she used to describe a process of erosion; this erosion is the effect of chronic stressors on the lives of Black and Brown people.

The fundamental problem is that these chronic stressors occur repeatedly throughout their entire lifespan and thereby create a general, overall health *vulnerability*.

In an interview, Geronimus described the death of a friend's family member. That deceased person used to enjoy playing the game of *Jenga*. For Geronimus, playing *Jenga* was a metaphor for what happens in *weathering* — as she alluded to by saying:

> *"They pull out one piece at a time, and another piece and another piece, until you sort of collapse. You start losing pieces of your health and well-being, but you still try to go on as long as you can. Even if you're disabled, even if it's hard, that you have a certain tenacity and hope, and sense of collective responsibility whether that's for your family or community. But there's a point where enough pieces have been pulled out of you, that you can no longer withstand, and you collapse."* [2]

Here is the hard truth. Chronic health conditions do not uniformly impact all people living in the US. If you have a chronic disorder in the US, such as diabetes, asthma, or high blood pressure, you are far more likely to be a person who is African American, Latinx, or Native American.

In 2019, the percentage of the African American population in the US living with diabetes was 16%, compared to 12% for the white population.[3]

Since our bodies all have nearly the same physiological make-up, heart, circulatory system, and other organs, other factors than our genes and bad luck are contributing to the extreme level of health disparities.

These factors are the social circumstances of health, such as income level, access to healthcare services, zip code, racism, and discrimination.

Yep! I said it out loud. Racism and discrimination do make you sick, literally! Moreover, they are designed to worsen your health as a mechanism of control.

In a report titled *Ethnic Disparities in the Burden and Treatment of Asthma*, the *Asthma and Allergy Foundation of America*, the co-authors stated: "In the United States, the burden of asthma falls disproportionately on the Black and Hispanic—mainly Puerto Rican—populations and especially on minority children."[4]

While you may feel more susceptible to developing a chronic health disorder or dying earlier than someone who is non-white and a US resident, understanding how the social determinants of health impact you is one of the ways that you can act to protect your future health and that of your loved ones.

Meanwhile, for a reader of this book who is white, comprehending how enduring injustices based on "race" foster an intensified likelihood of health disorders can enable you to change this damaging "status quo" and promote better overall health for all Americans.

Understanding the Structure of this Book

This book is divided into four parts as follows. The first part is focused predominantly on the most "studied" social determinants of health—nearly all of which are widely recognized by public health professionals as the major social factors of health.

The second part centers on related factors, such as the historically inappropriate medical care in the US for African American, Latinx, and Native American people and biased beliefs of healthcare providers.

For example, employment in the US is coupled to socioeconomic status, and socioeconomic status can be bonded to assumptions and predispositions of hospital and outpatient care employees.

In this way, there is a close relationship between the social determinants and factors described in Parts I and II in terms of the overall impact on the healthcare of Black and Brown people.

The third part of this book is focused on the specific impact of health insurance and the US health insurance industry as another social determinant of health. Part III also explores the effect of "high-deductible" health insurance on health status and health outcomes, as well as disparities in health status/health outcomes linked to Medicaid and Medicare coverage status.

In Part IV, the primary focus is *Health Justice* and advocating for equity in order to address race-based healthcare disparities. As mentioned, there is an overlap between the focus of these four parts.

For example, one chapter in this part is focused on the impact of the Covid-19 pandemic on Black and Brown people, since the fatality rate has been so disproportionately elevated, but Covid-19 is also discussed in earlier chapters as associated with a specific social determinant of health.

Essentially, each distinct part of this book discusses the given social element from a different vantage point as encompassed in that part. In this way, my goal is to enable you to acquire a broader understanding of the *scope* and interdependence of impact on health by each of the discussed factors.

The first chapter of this book concentrates on housing. This is because African Americans, Latinx people, and Native Americans have been most often steered to live in geographic areas in closer proximity to toxic levels of pollution and/or chemicals.

Whether through "redlining," in which banks denied mortgages to African Americans and all other Black and Brown people to purchase homes in all but specifically designated neighborhoods, or past urban development programs that "ghettoized" African American and Latinx people into specific zip codes, institutionalized racism has traditionally forced non-white US residents into housing that is more likely to be near toxic hazards—and, therefore, more unhealthy settings.

Meanwhile, the other chapters in Part I zone in on the other four primary areas in which Black and Brown people in the US have been deprived in terms of the social foundations interrelated to the overall quality of health.

From occupational choices to schools to grocery store options, social and behavioral patterns negatively impacting marginalized populations have contributed to disparities in overall health status between people considered white in the US and people of color.

As many of you probably know, these social determinants each adversely impact the health of African Americans, Latinx people, and Native Americans from birth onward.

Childhood is the time when a salubrious lifestyle is essential to prevent chronic disorders from developing, so altering the discrepancies in the social factors of health is crucial to enabling healthful lifestyles in all US children that will influence their well-being over a lifetime—and not just in privileged children.

The healthcare system in the US tends to benefit white patients, as well. Therefore, this book particularly includes chapters in Parts II and III that describe the diverse ways that healthcare clinician training programs, interactions between physicians and patients, hospital options for treatment, insurance companies, and various governmental healthcare policies hinder populations by ethnicity in the US.

Chapter 9 in Part II concentrates specifically on mental health and substance use disorders. Mental health impacts physical health, and systemic oppression in the US contributes to specific psychosocial outcomes in African American, Latinx, and Native American people in our nation.

Indeed, research study findings in *Psychiatric Services* revealed that "compared with non-Hispanic whites, African Americans and Hispanics report less access to mental health and substance use disorder treatment services and less utilization of and satisfaction with such services."[5]

Therefore, the impact of a lack of "culturally-competent" mental health and substance abuse disorder services is discussed in-depth in its own chapter.

My faith and beliefs are a couple of the things that ground my commitment to educating and empowering myself and others to live a wholesome lifestyle as one strategy of resistance to the race-based inequities of the US health system.

For this reason, Chapter 15 in Part IV includes a discussion of the role of faith leaders, nonprofit organizations, and community-based groups in advocating against inequities, particularly affecting the health and well-being of people of color.

Self-empowerment in terms of ending health incongruences includes advocating for change in the US, and recognition of the social determinants of health is the first step toward grasping the needed actions to reduce inequalities in overall health status in the US.

By understanding the effects of the various social determinants of health, you can be a better healthcare *advocate* for marginalized populations that are more likely to develop chronic disorders linked to a decreased quality of life.

Likewise, by building your knowledge base regarding the societal factors impacting overall health status, you can channel your energies more effectively as a healthcare activist, whether professional or volunteer, at eradicating the discriminations aimed at African American, Latinx, and Native American people that impact health and mortality. Change for the better is possible!

UNDERSTANDING THE SOCIAL DETERMINANTS OF HEALTH

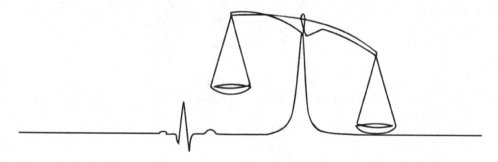

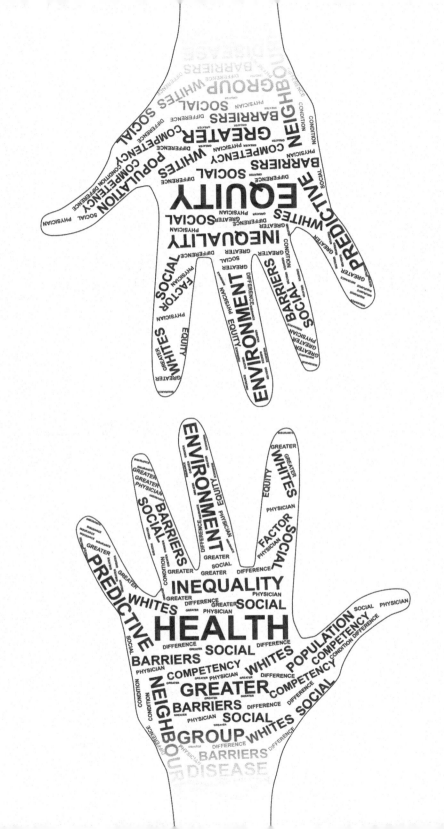

CHAPTER 1

Δ

HOUSING—IMPLICATIONS FOR HEALTH

I begin this chapter with a story to illustrate how something not directly related to health can impact overall medical care. Please bear with me. There was a lady—let's call her Destiny—and she was diagnosed with breast cancer.

At her oncologist's recommendation, Destiny agreed to undergo a double mastectomy to reduce the likelihood that the cancer would spread. After several weeks of testing, lab results, and office visits, she was scheduled for a double mastectomy.

On the morning of Destiny's procedure, the medical team expected her arrival, but she never showed up for surgery. The surgeon was extremely annoyed and felt his precious time that could have been utilized for someone else had been "wasted."

Not only did he consider Destiny non-compliant, inconsiderate, and lacking the appropriate sense of urgency around her care, but he decided that since she clearly did not care about her own health, he did not plan to reschedule with her.

Destiny was blessed, however! She had developed a great relationship with "Shelly," the Nurse Navigator, and Shelly knew that something had to be wrong for Destiny to fail to arrive for her surgery.

The following day after learning about this odd occurrence, Shelly contacted Destiny and discovered that she had received an eviction notice from her residence the evening prior to her appointment.

The impending eviction had created so much anxiety and fear for Destiny regarding how she and her children would survive that she did not have the mental fortitude to phone to cancel her surgery; instead, all of her vitality was absorbed into "survival mode."

Shelly understood that Destiny's top priority was safety and shelter for her children and herself, and not the breast cancer—even though *not* dealing with the breast cancer could result in additional dire consequences in the future.

To sum things up, Destiny decided not to have the bilateral mastectomy because she would be imminently living in her car, so how could she possibly recover following surgery or take care of herself while homeless?

As a proactive and caring nurse navigator, Shelly made a few phone calls to some community agencies and was able to help Destiny secure emergency housing, which eventually led to permanent housing.

Shelly also talked to the surgeon and explained the reason Destiny failed to phone to reschedule her procedure. Following Shelly's explanation, this surgeon felt a deep level of regret for his negative and bigoted attitude toward Destiny. Therefore, her surgery was rescheduled with them.

Instead of a horrific outcome, as occurs for so many marginalized and vulnerable people, Destiny ended on the path to recovery and in her new home.

If Shelly had not understood that some patients struggle with a complex spider web of external issues, leaving such basic needs as housing unmet, she would have viewed Destiny in an unfavorable light. I refer to this "complex spider's web" as *fighting poverty*.

The reason that I have begun this chapter with this story is for you to understand the following key point:

If you are both rich and white in the US, you are far more likely to have decent health and a longer lifespan than if you are not!

Intersectionality was coined by Kimberlee Crenshaw. A pioneering scholar and writer on civil rights, critical race theory, Black feminist legal theory, race, racism, and the law, Crenshaw wanted to create language to describe how sociological factors can overlap and heighten the disadvantages faced by an oppressed group.

In terms of African American, Latinx, and Native American people, the intersectionality of diverse disadvantages drives the profound inconsistencies reflected in overall health and mortality. In other words, if you are both rich and white in the US, you are *far* more likely to have decent health and a longer lifespan than if you are not!

Social determinants of health are conditions in the environments in which people are born, live, learn, work, play, worship, and age that affect a wide range of health, functioning, and quality of life outcomes and risks.

There is a range of factors that influence the health status of individuals or populations. It is noteworthy that only 10% of the elements of population health are attributed to the medical care, yet this is the predominant focus of medical care.

90% of population health foundations are linked to behavior, lifestyle, social circumstances, and environmental exposure. Thus, the circumstances in which we live explain in part why some Americans are healthier than others and why some Americans more generally are not.

Housing is so important to health that early humans around 300,000 years ago began living in caves to escalate their likelihood of survival. No doubt you already know that housing discrimination historically existed against African American people in the US as a legacy of slavery.

The early Jim Crow Era and the rising dominance of the Ku Klux Klan (KKK) during the first quarter of the 20th century so perpetuated African Americans living in life-threatening conditions that a mass migration of southern-born African Americans to Ohio, Illinois, and Michigan commenced.

This expanded to most Northern cities by the end of World War II.[6] Meanwhile, western agriculture depended primarily on Latinx farmworkers who were often housed on their employers' farms. As for Native Americans, they had been largely forced to live on reservations where access to water was limited.

While low-income white people also had fewer choices when it came to housing options, race-based laws restricted people of color into living spaces that were simply bad for health.

The necessity of adequate housing is so essential to child health and development—and to preventing the development of chronic disorders impacting every aspect of life—that this is the reason the *first* chapter in this book is focused on housing as a social determinant of health.

Home Ownership as an Aspect of the American Dream — Why a Home Matters

The practice of *redlining* is defined in the dictionary as "refusing to offer credit or insurance in a particular community on a discriminatory basis."[7]

Author Richard Rothstein noted in *The Color of Law* that federal housing programs beginning in the 1930s promoted "state-sponsored segregation" through redlining.[8]

Owning a home has always been a path for US residents to build wealth and credit. If you are unable to obtain a mortgage or credit, it is hard to climb the ladder of wealth-building.

The gap in homeownership in the US is clear in that the African American homeownership rate was 41% in 2017, compared to a white homeownership rate of 72% (and this ownership divergence has grown by 30% since 2010).[9]

In addition to difficulty in attaining financing to purchase or maintain a home (or condo), in neighborhoods where Black and Brown people have purchased homes have most often led to "white flight" with a resultant decrease in property values (the re-sale value of that home). This problem still exists today.

In 2017, I decided to go for a walk in my own neighborhood that happens to be predominantly white. While walking, I held my (at the time) six-month-old grandson in my arms. Just blocks from my home that I own, a driver slowed down his vehicle as he rode along.

He then leaned from the window to yell at me, "Get out of our neighborhood, Nigger." I was in complete shock and disgust but digressed to tell you about this personal experience so you can grasp the present-day effect of historical "redlining" on the everyday lives of Black and Brown people.

Renting an apartment or house that someone else owns aids in paying off the *owner's* mortgage rather than building equity. All too often, rental units occupied by Black and Brown people are in geographic locations that enable proximity to pollutants, pathogenic bacteria, and other hazards.

Never mind considering the price-gouging grocery stores, the poor schools, and the shoddy housing construction. Whether rural or urban, the housing available to Black and Brown people has been worse than that available to the white population.

Cancer Rate — The Link to Housing

African Americans comprise only 13% of the total US population but have the shortest survival rate and the greatest death rate from cancer of any ethnic group in the US, per the American Cancer Society.[10]

Besides lower access to healthcare services than other populations in the US, inadequate housing contributes to this problem. Drinking and bathing water contaminants are particularly associated with cancer development in children.

Since some abnormal tumors can take decades to become cancerous, the toxic hazards that babies and children are exposed to contribute to their likelihood of having cancer in adulthood.

The National Cancer Institute remarks that nitrate run-off is especially *carcinogenic* (cancer-causing),[11] and this byproduct of large-scale agriculture especially affects African American, Latinx, and Native American people in rural areas.

Leukemia (acute lymphocytic leukemia [ALL]) is the most common cancer diagnosed in children, constituting 25% of all childhood cancers.[12]

In Jonathan Harr's book, *A Civil Action*, in 1996, a lawsuit resulted in a judgment against companies enabling toxic run-off to enter drinking and bathing water related to a leukemia "cluster" in nearby communities.[13]

In 2015, the prominent lead level in the drinking water of Flint, MI (that was both recognized and hidden by state government officials) was publicly exposed by Dr. Mona Hanna-Attisha; she documented her experience of activism to improve Flint's drinking water quality in her book, *What the Eyes Don't See*.[14]

Lead—whether carried in the water through rusted pipes or absorbed through skin as a component of paint used in a home—is poisonous and linked to neurological disorders, including brain tumors.

Poor children are more likely to encounter lead exposure than children of elevated socioeconomic backgrounds due to the greater likelihood of old pipes and lead-containing paint (now banned for use by the US Consumer Product Safety Commission).

While asbestos—concurrent to lung dysfunction—is similarly banned, it still exists in the basements of many older homes.

Outdated housing stock in run-down condition is most often the type available for ownership or rental by Black and Brown people.

Meanwhile, the neighborhoods with this housing tend to have less governmental monies allotted for sanitation—enabling more illnesses and infections to thrive and worse air quality due to a raised likelihood of nearby manufacturing facilities (not "zoned" for inclusion in white neighborhoods) emitting fumes into the air.

Public Housing as a Social Determinant of Health

The purpose of federally funded (and state-funded) public housing was to provide housing for the poor. According to the US Dept. of Housing and Urban Development (HUD), around one point two million households in the US live in federally funded public housing.[15]

In order to qualify for a rental unit in public housing, you have to meet a poverty threshold so low that you were probably unable to pay for any "out-of-pocket" healthcare costs not covered by insurance.

In the US, the poverty rate in 2018 was 9% for white residents but 22% for African Americans, 19% for Latinx/Hispanics, and 24% for Native Americans.[16]

However, only 48% of public housing occupants were Black or Brown.[17] Nobody *wants* to live in public housing because the rental units tend to be run-down and located in areas inconvenient to shopping, workplaces, houses of worship, and other facilities usual to a community.

The main reason for the lack of close access to facilities that aid in community-building are state and local zoning ordinances that preserve the status quo. Therefore, it can take a Herculean effort to change the foundational elements of communities to help residents of a neighborhood feel pride in their community based on zip code.

Urban Renewal — Impact on Black and Brown Communities

The resilience of communities of color is demonstrated by the creation of thriving neighborhoods despite policies and laws designed to prevent non-white residents from achieving fairness in the areas associated with the social determinants of health, of which housing is only one.

Yet, historical records indicate these thriving communities have emerged despite the odds stacked against them.

The *Housing Act* of 1949 under President Truman became the legal basis for purchasing African-American-owned homes at low prices to tear them down for the ostensible purpose of rebuilding the area with better-quality housing stock and neighborhood layout.

What actually happened was that thriving neighborhoods were demolished, and people of color were forced to relocate out of their community.

75% of the people impacted by urban renewal projects were people of color. In San Francisco in the 1950s, the Western Edition/Fillmore neighborhood was wiped out (requiring the relocation of 20,000 people), but nothing was rebuilt for decades.[18]

When the reconstruction finally occurred, white occupants and business owners purchased the new properties. This urban demolition and shifting of property ownership were repeated in big cities across the US.

No wonder communities of color face such tremendous obstacles in accomplishing change that fundamentally alters the status quo when it comes to achieving socioeconomic equality in the US! Yes, systematic shenanigans for the win!

How People in the US Perceive Their Housing and Communities

The inequity in housing has generated a vastly divided perspective on housing and community between the white and non-white populations, according to findings of a national study in 2018 of the nonprofit Pew Research Center.

In suburban and rural areas, the white residents were far more satisfied with their lives in their community than the non-white residents. However, 59% of all respondents felt some attachment to their local community, and 81% of respondents who reported knowing all (or most) of their neighbors expressed attachment to the area.

Meanwhile, 65% of homeowners communicated feelings of attachment as opposed to only 52% of renters. One of the conclusions stated in this Pew Research Center report is that "family ties draw many people back to the place they grew up." [19]

Indeed, this may be a reason—besides socioeconomic factors—why people remain in housing and communities that negatively impact their quality of life.

Uranium Mining Waste and Native American Communities

Uranium mining sponsored by the US Department of Energy for use by nuclear power plants and the military occurred near Native American reservations. The radiation-emitting waste from these mining operations was not identified as toxic to nearby residents, and the result was a huge radiation exposure to Native American children.

The US Indian Health Service (IHS) is charged with providing healthcare services to Native Americans residing on the reservations but has generally provided limited access to patient care.

Meanwhile, a medical research article published in 2017 noted that proximity to the uranium mines was connected to a higher prevalence of kidney disease and numerous other disorders.[20]

The presentation of this information is for recognition that while there are similarities in housing inequity between Brown and Black populations linked to the promotion of chronic disorders, differences in health effects also exist.

Focus on Asthma — The Housing Connection

The prevalence of asthma is augmented among African Americans but even greater among Latinx people—especially Puerto Ricans. Nearly 17% of all Puerto Ricans in the US have asthma, and Puerto Ricans are the most prone to undergo a fatal asthma attack.[21]

Moreover, Puerto Ricans tend to live in dense urban housing, with nearly 94% living in urban settings in Puerto Rico[22] and nearly the same percent in urban environments on the US mainland (primarily in cities in New York and Florida).

The overall poverty level for Puerto Ricans is high, and this has forced an extraordinary percentage of Puerto Rican families to reside in substandard housing.

Additionally, crowded living conditions with intergenerational households all living under the same roof contribute to weak indoor air quality.

Most Puerto Ricans in the US mainland live in New York City, particularly in the Bronx (which is predominantly Latinx).

Cockroach waste, rat feces, and dust—which are all associated with an enhanced risk for asthma—are rampant in lower-income neighborhoods in New York City. Even in the small city of Springfield, MA, asthma is highest in the Puerto Rican population!

A foremost problem supplementary with asthma starting in childhood is that the more asthma episodes in nonage, the higher the chance of severe asthma in adulthood.

Since Black and Brown people are more susceptible to develop asthma in their youth (with a link to low-quality housing) and are less likely to be able to access first-rate and culturally sensitive medical care when needed, the probability of disabling chronic asthma in adulthood is increased—thereby, fostering a vicious cycle for the families impacted by asthma.

As a social determinant of health, housing is at the top of the list because of its ability to foster this brutal cycle, leading to worsening overall health outcomes.

Anyone who wonders why a person of color in this situation does not just move their family somewhere else does not understand the factors preventing residential relocation to promote better health and well-being.

Homelessness also disproportionately affects Black and Brown people, and "dumping" homeless people into substandard housing is not an acceptable solution to the problem.

Here is the real deal. The institutionalized racism underpinning housing options for non-white people in the US has been the main obstacle preventing expanded access to health-boosting housing by African American, Latinx, and Native American families.

Thus, public health measures to reduce health gaps between white US residents and everyone else need to address the housing disparity and systematic racism that fuels it through micro-aggressive and discriminatory laws, policies, guidelines, and regulations.

I'd like to pause here to talk further about systematic racism and microaggressions. There is a misconception that a specific group of individuals working within a particular field (*e.g.*, healthcare) is intrinsically racist.

However, the totality of the ways in which US society fosters the acceptance of narrow-minded institutional policies, procedures, guidelines, and practices may produce interpersonal conflict rather than some type of personally held racist belief on the part of everyone in that given field.

My purpose in writing this is so that you consider that a racist statement or action may not be intentional but nevertheless result in the same racist outcome.

Microaggressions can be unintentional. They often involve hostile and/or derogatory communications or attitudes directed toward marginalized populations. Similar to the misery caused by living each day with a myriad of disadvantages that create obstacles for the affected people, small microaggressions can add up to a 12,000-foot mountain over time.

Metaphorically speaking, this can cause Black and Brown people to face a Mount Everest of microaggressions on a daily basis.

For example, being profiled while shopping, being mistaken as a janitor in the hospital when you are a physician, being pulled over by police officers while driving through a predominately white neighborhood in a nice car, being told your articulation is professional, being mistaken for a valet at a black-tie event while waiting for your car.

The list goes on and on. And, yes, it does get frustrating and tiring!

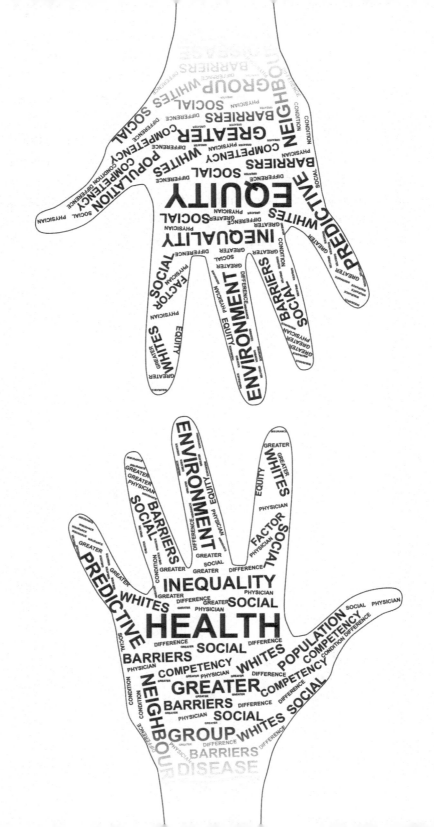

CHAPTER 2

Δ

EDUCATION AND SCHOOLING

The US Supreme Court decision in *Brown v. Board of Education* (five cases heard in 1954-1955)[23] was considered the landmark court ruling desegregating public schools.

We know that this did not actually happen, partly due to the ruling's vague language that did not specify how this desegregation would occur.

Meanwhile, the term *affirmative action* was coined by African American lawyer, Hobart Taylor, Jr. chosen by President Lyndon Johnson to chair a committee promoting equal rights for minorities,[24] and culminating in the passage of Johnson's *Civil Rights Act*, legislating affirmative action in employment.

In the years following *Brown v. Board of Education*, African American parents began to demand improved educational opportunities for their children even more insistently.

Indeed, some Black and Brown kids were able to get a better education one way or another. Then in 1978, the US Supreme Court ruled the use of quotas to accomplish the goals of affirmative action as unconstitutional.[25]

Next, in the 1990s, affirmative action laws began to be overturned nationwide. Instead of affirmative action, the catchphrase became *diversity*. But unlike affirmative action, diversity did not have the weight of any legislation to enforce it.

This is the condensed historical account of how African American youth became permitted to attend white schools and universities that had formerly prevented their admission.

However, this book is about social imbalances in healthcare and not US history, so this description sums up the "two steps forward, one step back" in terms of equal educational access that has occurred over the past sixty years.

The School Graduation Rate Disparity and What
This Means for Healthcare Access

Per the National Center for Education Statistics, the domestic graduation rate for all high school enrollees in the 2017-2018 school year was 85%. Of these high school students, the Latinx graduation rate was 81%, African American 79%, and white 89%.[26]

It is nearly impossible for anyone without a high school diploma to acquire any type of employment now. In the 1980s, a high school diploma was sufficient for an administrative assistant or data entry job.

No longer. More and more post-high school degrees and certificates seem to be needed to acquire entry-level white-collar jobs. Presently, nearly all employers for low-level white-collar jobs require candidates to hold a four-year college degree. This has also become the case in the past twenty years for employment in the manufacturing sector!

The disparity among college graduates based on race is even wider. Among solely public colleges in 2013, the overall graduation rate was 63%, but the African American graduation rate was 47%, paralleled to 65% for white attendees.[27]

The two primary factors underpinning this difference are the overall lower quality of K-12 schools that Black and Brown children attend, combined with the lack of financial resources on the part of non-white parents to pay for the ever-increasing college tuition of their offspring.

This, by far, is not the whole story, but it leaves Black and Brown youth at a significant disadvantage when it comes to acquiring an education.

If you do not have the educational attainment to acquire a well-paying job, chances are you will not be able to acquire quality health insurance through your job or by purchasing it yourself, such as a plan with a low annual deductible and/or low co-pays.

If enrolled in a high-deductible health plan (*i.e.*, one that requires $1,000 or more out-of-pocket before health coverage begins), a young adult is far more prone to skip visits to a healthcare facility for basic preventive care—ditto for early detection with most forms of cancer.

Meanwhile, a lower literacy level (reading ability) can make it difficult to understand health education brochures (health literacy) and the instructional inserts accompanying both prescription drugs and over-the-counter medicines.

Not to mention reading and signing *Informed Consent* forms nationally required by hospitals before surgery, inclusion in clinical trials, or other treatments/diagnostic tests. Also, health education printed materials and online resources geared to educated readers can be overwhelming for someone with only a high school education!

I'm sure you have read some type of health education material with complex medical terminology that was impossible to comprehend! Despite attempts to simplify the language of health education material, much healthcare information, especially brochures and online hand-outs, can be utterly confusing to most people.

Inequities in School Funding and Resources

Predominantly African American and Latinx-enrolled schools have historically received far less funding from federal, state, and local governments.

Since the most significant proportion of funds for schools comes from local sources, the generally lower socioeconomic status interconnected to African American and Latinx neighborhoods translates into lower tax dollars and property tax revenue to fund the neighborhood's schools.

The poorer the neighborhood, the less local government money for schools. The wealthier the community, the more money available to rehabilitating a school building (or replacing it with a new one), as well as everything else targeted at enriching students' experiences and enjoyment of public school.

I have firsthand experience with this issue that occurred while my son was a sophomore in high school. During a parent-teacher conference, my son's pre-algebra teacher informed me that textbooks were not in the school budget.

How can students thrive without textbooks as reference material, especially when it comes to math? The answer to this rhetorical question is that such a situation makes it that much more difficult for the kids!

Fact: the end result for schools disproportionately serving Black and Brown kids is that schools tend to be in worse condition (inclusive of more environmental hazards) and have larger class sizes than in white schools.

> *How can students thrive without textbooks as reference material, especially when it comes to math? The answer to this rhetorical question is that such a situation makes it that much more difficult for the kids!*

Meanwhile, school libraries, enrichment programs, media and technology access, and school-supplied materials tend to be more limited in predominantly African American, Latinx, and Native American-enrolled schools.

Similar to the Industrial Revolution, it is important to recognize how major the global workforce shift has been toward relying on high-level information technology (IT) skills.

In fact, IT access is even more significant as workplaces, since the 1990s have required an ever-increasing knowledge level of high-tech software programs and computer hardware.

The current Covid-19 pandemic creates an additional burden for students without reliable internet connectivity and up-to-date notebook computers, as schools and colleges have shifted to online learning to prevent transmission of the virus.

This requires the ability to download and utilize teleconferencing software platforms (inclusive of video and audio components) to interact in real-time with teachers and other students.

When this pandemic is over, it is doubtful that schools will return to not incorporate online learning as teachers adapt to fashioning their lesson plans to interact with students off-site.

Impoverished families that cannot afford to purchase the technology necessary will be placed at an even more severe disadvantage in acquiring a favorable education for their offspring.

The educational achievement gap based on economic status is estimated to be widened in the coming years, so this definitely needs to be addressed well before it becomes the new reality!

Bias in Course Content and Testing — Impact on Black and Brown Students

The social studies and English course content in most public schools across the country can leave a student thinking that the history of the world (and all critically esteemed authors) have been solely white people's achievements.

The true history of Black and Brown people in the US has been utterly revised to stress the contributions of white people—including the roles of white people to better the lives of the non-white population.

Instead of learning about the vital contributions of Frederick Douglas, Charlotte Forten Grimke, and W.E.B. DuBois, high school students learn about Lewis and Clark expeditions and various generals who oversaw numerous wars.

Furthermore, many of the written works by these historical figures and/or fiction authors are steeped in racist opinions of Black and Brown people.

The SATs and GREs have been focal measures to determine an applicant's worthiness for acceptance into an undergraduate collegiate program and graduate school, respectively.

Yet, these both incorporate biases toward familiarity with white history and famous books, as well as written English based on a thorough understanding of the King's English of the *Oxford Dictionary*. Therefore, scholastic testing has been another manner by which Black and Brown youth have been deprived.

And then, there is the matter of financial resources to contribute to the education of a family's children from nursery school to college graduation.

Youth from socioeconomically privileged backgrounds are far more apt to have paid tutors in school courses difficult for them and attend afterschool classes to prepare them to take SATs, GREs, and other tests (such as the MCAT for medical school admission or LSAT for law school admission).

As if this was not enough of an obstacle to acquiring a suitable education, guidance counselors in K-12 schools are more likely to steer Black and Brown youth toward a lower level of career aspiration.

It should be no surprise that so many African American, Latinx, and Native American youth end up not trying to acquire the higher education necessary for a career as a physician, lawyer, professor, or engineer.

Lack of Teacher/Professor Role Models and its Effect

The US National Center for Education Statistics (*NCES*) notes that out of the one and a half million faculty members in 2017 in degree-granting post-secondary schools, 41% were white males and 35% were white females. In contrast, 3% were African American or Latinx, and an even tinier percentage were Native American.[28]

In elementary schools and high schools, most teachers are white, whether in predominantly white schools or minority schools.

For schools that are disproportionately composed of Black and/or Brown students, the teachers are typically less well-trained, whether white or non-white and/or earlier in their teaching careers, and therefore paid a lower salary.

The lower salary level is why teachers working in impoverished schools tend to rotate annually and/or leave the K-12 education field altogether, rather than enable students to have the consistency in their school's teachers common to schools in high-income communities.

The lack of role models in the classroom can leave minority students discouraged about their future opportunities in life.

In turn, this can result in a lessened interest in school achievement. A lack of college education among the parents and grandparents of these youth is another obstacle to acquiring the grades necessary to succeed in high school and college.

Ponder this question—what year in school did you experience having your first Black or Brown teacher? What about a Black male? I was in the final semester of my master's program.

This is because under-educated parents do not have the academic knowledge level to assist their offspring in understanding challenging school assignments (such as developing the underlying argument of a research paper) compared to college-educated parents.

For the children of parents who attended college, the road to advancing their own education has far fewer potholes.

Naturally, they are more able to craft essays for admission to colleges that display a broader depth of extracurricular participation (*e.g.*, participating in the school's track team or orchestra), plus participating in a year-abroad study program.

Lack of Opportunity for Extracurricular Activities

Volunteering for a year after school each day in a hospital sounds far more impressive to college admission reviewers than "worked every day after school delivering pizzas or washing cars."

However, working jobs such as above is necessary for many low-income youths aspiring to attend a prestigious university, especially if they are transferring from a two-year community college.

Even for students that do complete college with the intent of entering the healthcare field, attending a less respected medical or nursing school can result in expanded difficulties in gaining a residency placement *after* finishing school or entering a more substantially paid hospital nursing specialty as a "new nurse" (*e.g.*, as a Newborn Intensive Care Unit [NICU] or Cardiology Care Unit [CCU] nurse).

I am by no means implying that the possibility of successful advancement does not exist, but in many cases, the opportunities are far less readily attainable for marginalized populations.

Public Schools Unraveling—How "Bad" Schools
Lead to the Growth of Alternative Models

The first charter school in the US opened in 1992. Since then, the charter school movement has exploded.[29] Charter schools are taxpayer-funded public schools that are alternatives to typical public K-12 schools.

The basis for acceptance of a high-achieving student is through a lottery system, so most qualified students are not accepted into their targeted charter school. Instead, the non-chosen students typically attend their local public school.

Yes, the selection process is much like a casino lottery. There are always more losers than winners in this type of selection process. For the winners, a charter school education can be the ticket to an excellent learning experience at no greater cost than attendance at a public school.

Charter schools across the nation have been embraced as a positive step by a hefty proportion of society, but the funding for these schools comes out of the state budgets for public schools (and some of these schools can discriminate in hiring staff more readily than public schools, due to different regulations governing their administration).

Meanwhile—since the Latinx population is disproportionately Catholic—many Latinx families who can afford it prefer a parochial education for their children.

Beginning in 2017, the problem of underfunding public schools was tremendously exacerbated by President Trump's choice for his Secretary of Education, Betsy DeVos.

DeVos was a vociferous opponent of public-school education even before she was appointed, as well being a supporter of for-profit, vocational, post-secondary schools (that are expensive and especially attracted to Black and Latinx students for enrollment, but without leading to the promised jobs after completion). Therefore, much progress for disadvantaged youth was reversed during her tenure.

According to the Pennsylvania Education Association (PEA), as Secretary of Education, Devos invoked her authority to no longer enforce provisions requiring federally funded education services to be provided by public employees.

This made it so private schools and religious-affiliated schools could receive funding previously reserved for public education across the country. In addition, she cut public school funding by $8.5 billion in 2020, including eliminating most of the federal budget for teacher development programs, academic support and enrichment, and afterschool activities.[30]

Meanwhile, she repealed the Obama Administration's regulation closing for-profit, post-secondary, and vocational schools that perpetrated fraud against Black and Brown students through providing high-interest loans based on false promises of future job placement.[31]

Similarly, the PEA also reports that this Secretary of Education was a strong supporter of President Trump's plan to eliminate the Public Service Loan Forgiveness Program. Hopefully, these changes will be reversed under our new administration!

It is vital to realize that professional, middle-class, white parents historically have more easily sent their children and teenagers to better schools when they perceived the neighborhood school to be sub-optimal for their offspring.

In contrast, this has been astronomically harder for Black and Brown parents (as well as for Native Americans, who have the most notable high school drop-out rate of any ethnic group in the US[32]).

In other words, the "wiggle-room" for getting a good education to enter a chosen profession is significantly narrower for people in the US who are not upper-middle-class and white.

Disparities in the Healthcare Workforce Linked to Education

Most physicians and registered nurses in the US are white, which probably comes as no surprise. Per the Association of American Medical Colleges (AAMC), only 5.8% of all physicians in the US in 2018 were Latinx/Hispanic, 5% were African American, and 17.1% were Asian.[33]

Meanwhile, medical research studies have shown that African Americans have a larger tendency than other ethnic groups to distrust white medical providers due to the historical mistreatment of Black people by the US medical system,[34] such as occurred during the federal Tuskegee Experiment, and the forced sterilization of African American women (We will learn more about this in Part II).

Particularly among Latinx people, a lack of English language fluency and/or cultural barriers can reduce the trust of white healthcare providers.

For example, dermatologists are trained to diagnose skin infections and possible cancers on white skin.

According to *Social Science and Medicine*, "even though medical texts often have overall proportional racial representation, this is not the case for skin tone. Furthermore, racial minorities are still often absent at the topic level."

Black skin only appears in 4.5% of medical books. This leads to many gaps for people of color.[35]

Inflammation on someone with dark skin will not show as red as it does on pale skin, leading doctors to believe the issue is more minimal than it truly is. Another example is the myth that Black people have a higher pain tolerance than other races.

As *The Proceedings of the National Academy of Sciences* states, "Black Americans are systematically undertreated for pain relative to white Americans." [36]

This racial bias kills patients and furthers mistrust in the doctor-patient relationship.

Black, Brown, and Asian immigrants all tend to face issues related to a lack of cultural competence among white doctors, and such a lack of trust can lead to them foregoing needed healthcare and/or not complying with doctor's orders and returning for essential follow up care.

The intense competition for medical school admission has long favored applicants who attended expensive ivy league universities and achieved high MCAT scores.

On top of that, the cost of medical school is frequently out of reach for college students with limited financial resources. However, the historical ramifications of this disparity for the medical care provided to Black and Brown people have been, and remains, simply enormous.

Link Between Literacy and Health Quality

The inability to seek and understand health information in the US is especially difficult for people with low literacy levels and/or those who are not fluent in the English language.

Medical terminology can be another obstacle to comprehension for people attempting to read informative brochures and books on specific health disorders. Likewise, it is far easier for someone with a low literacy level to be scammed by unscrupulous snake oil manufacturers promising miracle cures.

And that's just a brief introduction to the problems facing people with low literacy levels in protecting their health. If you do not understand how your body works, it is far more difficult for you to understand why you may need to make a lifestyle change to preserve your health or undergo diagnostic tests such as an MRI or CAT scan.

Consequently, people with low educational attainment levels are far more likely to not seek early cancer treatment, change eating habits to lower cholesterol levels, and/or recognize the danger of not addressing persistently high blood pressure or uncontrolled diabetes.

They are far more likely to not know if they are being mistreated by an inexperienced doctor or one with a revoked license to practice medicine or to ask questions regarding options for treating a particular condition (*i.e.,* whether a minimally invasive surgery is available rather than surgery necessitating a sizable incision and numerous stitches).

The key takeaway in this chapter is that historical discrimination in education has led to increased obstacles for Black and Brown people to obtain a formidable education that is crucial for not only a better job with higher pay but also for receiving reputable healthcare services.

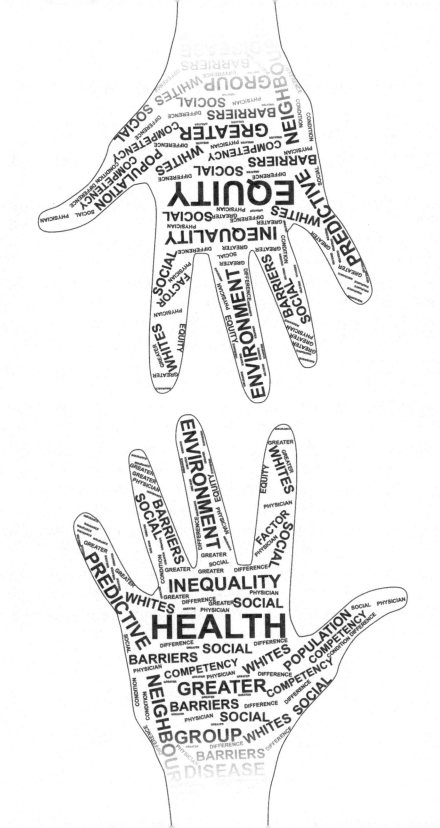

CHAPTER 3

Δ

WORK/EMPLOYMENT

Y ou are probably aware of the inequality in employment that affects the daily lives of African American, Latinx, and Native American people. As a nation founded upon slavery, an underclass of workers remains the backbone of the nation's economic engine.

Title VII of the *Civil Rights Act* of 1964 legally rendered discrimination based on employment illegal. However, employers get around this law by pretending that the reason a person of color was not hired was merely due to a lack of skills and/or they say a different applicant had more desired qualifications.

While a few employers annually are charged with violating anti-discrimination laws, many get away with it and go unpunished.

What Caste Has to Do with Discrimination in Employment

India has a 2,000-year-old caste system that was ostensibly abolished in 1950. However, it is well-recognized that *Dalits* (also called untouchables) remain economically at the bottom of the societal ladder. Somewhat better off than *Dalits*, *Shudras* (the fourth-lowest caste) are largely day-laborers, while *Vaishyas* (the third-lowest caste) are primarily merchants.

Although India's law regarding caste has enabled some socioeconomic improvement and much broader options for *Shudras* and *Vaishyas* (who are descendants of people performing similar work roles), *Dalits* are still the victims of society-wide contempt, creating no viable path for their employment or improved social status. Thus, *Dalits* remain mostly beggars and are indiscriminately victimized throughout India.

The idea of the US being a classless society has been promoted in our educational system to maintain the status quo, but a caste system (inclusive of socioeconomic class as an element) is evident in the US to people who are impoverished and not white.

You have only to consider who is most likely to work in the meat-packing plants and agricultural fields of large-scale *AgriBusiness* farms to recognize this invisible caste system.

Undocumented Mexican and Central American workers are the employees favored by these industries due to their willingness to work long hours for low pay and also to live in terrible conditions without complaining for fear of losing their employment and probable deportation.

How Covid-19 is Increasing Awareness of "Essential Workers"

The Covid-19 pandemic is shining a spotlight on essential workers. These are US labor force members who, while at greatest risk of Covid-19 infection, must go to work each day for society to function.

Besides doctors, nurses, and allied health professionals (*e.g.*, physical therapists), essential workers comprise grocery store clerks, gas station attendants, sanitation workers, custodians, bus drivers, home healthcare aides, housekeepers, and other "non-skilled" workers that enable US society to function smoothly.

African Americans, Latinx people, and first-generation immigrants are most likely to work in roles commonly devalued but now called "essential." Ironically, these low-paid workers are often not provided any health insurance coverage by their employers, never mind a regular work-week schedule, sick days, or vacation time.

While non-skilled essential workers may be identified right now as heroes (along with healthcare professionals) during this pandemic, that designation does not seem to have resulted in augmented pay or respect for their work. It is also no coincidence that Black and Brown people are over-represented in these under-valued and scantily-paid work roles.

If you have ever spent much time in a medical center environment, it is one of the most color-coded workplaces in the US. While most of the high-paid, professional employees are white, the frontline and lowest-paid staff are predominantly Black or Brown.

Who says there is no caste system in the US? The difference between India and the US is that members of India's society acknowledge there is a caste system. In contrast, our society's most privileged members do not recognize its plain-as-day existence in the US.

This denial can have particularly damaging effects on the self-esteem of everyone in the US not in the upper-middle and "owning" classes due to an increased risk for self-blame linked to an inability to overcome the obstacles generated by the supposedly nonexistent caste status.

It really is not your fault if you feel that you are too often just banging your head against the wall as you struggle to achieve the "American Dream."

Considering the "Direct Care" Workforce

According to a research brief in 2018, the direct care workforce includes 4.5 million personal care aides, home health aides, and nursing assistants. From 2005-2015, Black and African American women nationwide made up around 30% of this workforce, and Latinx women were also substantially represented.

Meanwhile, this same research brief noted, "Compared to white workers and Black immigrants in direct care [jobs], US-born Black/African American direct care workers are more prone to live in poverty and rely on public assistance."[37]

In many east coast cities, direct care workers in nursing homes are frequently Haitian immigrants. Nursing homes often did not have enough Personal Protective Equipment (PPE) in the early months of the Covid-19 pandemic, contrasted with hospitals, whose supplies were limited as well, but the disparity for nursing homes was far worse.

Since nursing homes have the overall uppermost Covid-19 infection rates (and fatality rates), these essential workers are at an incredible risk of becoming infected themselves and then infecting their family members and friends.

Implications of Low Educational Attainment on Employment and Hourly Wage

Only 6% of African Americans (aged twenty-five and older) in the US workforce had less than a high school diploma in 2018, and 31% had at least a bachelor's degree.[38]

As previously mentioned, it is nearly impossible for someone without a high school diploma to acquire a job in today's market.

Meanwhile, even possessing a bachelor's degree does not necessarily enable entry into a professional career with an hourly wage sufficient to save for retirement.

Low educational attainment adds a burden on African American, Latinx, and Native American people in the labor force as it can be used as justification for paying a lower wage than paid to an employee with a higher level of educational attainment *performing the same job*.

The problem is that people of color are disproportionately steered toward lower-paid employment and away from supervisorial positions. This is the "soft bigotry" of low expectations. Consequently, people of color in the labor force tend to be unable to improve socioeconomic status as much as their white counterparts.

Inequities in the Workplace Targeting Black and Brown People

Study findings from the Pew Research Center showed that African Americans, on average, earned 75% as much as whites in median hourly earnings as of 2015.[39]

The racial earnings gap appears to be narrowing, although the economic downturn (as a consequence of the Covid-19 pandemic) may reverse the recent gains. This *Pew* study also showed that white men out-earn African American and Latinx men, and all ethnicities of women.

An additional finding was that white and Asian women have narrowed the wage gap with white men to a much greater extent than African American or Latinx women.

Whether in a nonprofessional or professional position, whites are typically paid more than Black or Brown employees. It is also much harder for Black and Brown employees to advance and, thereby, earn a loftier income as well as more respect for their contributions.

According to the National Partnership for Women and Families in 2020, women of color encounter the nation's persistent and pervasive gender wage gap most severely.

Their recent report, *Quantifying America's Gender Wage Gap by Race/Ethnicity*, notes that Latinx females are typically paid just fifty-four cents for every dollar paid to a white male, and Native American females generally are paid just fifty-seven cents for every dollar given to a white male.

Meanwhile, African American females are paid just sixty-two cents for every dollar given to a white male, while white females are typically paid seventy-nine cents for every dollar given to a white male.[40]

This inequity is not just unfair. It has the potential to prevent anyone but white men from achieving the level of wealth that equates to power in our society.

At that time I began writing this book there were 615 billionaires in the US, and only six are African American.[41]

While economic inequality is widening in the US *(such that more billionaires are emerging even as more Americans are living in poverty)*, this outrageous statistic still demonstrates injustice between the white US population and the African American population.

This is yet another example of how systemic racism prevents Black and Brown people from accessing more societal power for self-determination.

There are 615 billionaires in the US, and only six are African American.

The amount of money available for investing, purchasing a home, paying for children's college education, or starting a small business venture to the under-earning woman is really stolen dollars.

It is the funds that cannot be used to donate to a nonprofit organization aiding Black and Brown women, jump-starting a community-based organization to improve neighborhood conditions, and/or political candidates supporting governmental policies addressing race-based inequities.

In other words, it is the wealth that white men acquire that supports the continuation of the status quo in terms of inequality. This leg up is denied to everyone who is not a white man.

CHAPTER 4

Δ

TRANSPORTATION ACCESS

Not having an automobile in a rural area of the US can mean not being able to show up for a healthcare appointment or hold a full-time job. However, unreliable public transportation in a suburban or urban area can create similar problems.

Meanwhile, the daily cost of gasoline, bus fare, and train fare can take a big bite out of a low-income worker's annual income, depending upon where that employee lives and works in the US.

For those that cannot relate to this difficulty, I recommend that you read the content of the website named "Asset Limited, Income Constrained, Employed (ALICE)" (www.unitedforalice.org) of the *United Way* of New Jersey.[42]

ALICE represents a way of defining and understanding the struggles of households with incomes above the Federal Poverty Level (FPL) but below a livable income for the geographic area in the US in which the home is located. In other words, it describes "the working poor."

I strongly recommend that you access the ALICE Poverty Simulator (developed by *Rebel Interactive Group* [https://Rebelinteractivegroup.com]). It is described on this website as an "interactive, engaging and easy to use mobile responsive, online experience that focuses on the population referred to as ALICE."[43]

This tool aims to make it to the end of the month without running out of money. Although it can sound simple, for a person living on the monthly wages of the "working poor," it is certainly not simple. This is why I encourage you to try this tool yourself!

Physicians tend to ignore, often unintentionally, transportation as a factor when determining a treatment plan for a patient based on their health problems. This is often overlooked by public health educators encouraging increased preventive care access, as well.

It is all wonderful to recommend that a woman obtain an annual mammogram, a person over age sixty-five receive a pneumonia vaccine injection, a newly diagnosed diabetic get nutrition counseling, and/or a smoker attend a smoking cessation program. However, people have to be able to transport themselves to physicians (and allied health) providers' offices to acquire healthcare.

Overall, people fighting poverty take about three times as many transit trips as those in higher-income groups (according to a report by the Federal Highway Administration in 2014).

This report also notes that households with children tend to travel annually twice as much (in total miles) as those without children.[44]

Since people of color are disproportionately impoverished contrasted to the white population of the US, a lack of reliable transportation presents yet another social disparity affecting access to healthcare.

Why is Transportation Access Such a Problem in the US?

Not all wealthy nations consider transportation a non-governmental area of concern as it regards their residents. In England, you can take a bus or train to most villages and all urban areas.

This is not to say that the cost of this transportation is not expensive, but at least it exists. The widespread existence of trains as a mode of transportation in England occurred because Queen Victoria loved her first train ride in the mid-nineteenth century so much that she supported the development of a national railway network.

Therefore, three billion British pounds were spent between the years 1845 and 1900 on building railways. In 1870, 432 million people in England traveled on 16,000 miles of railway track.[45] A smaller proportion of people in England own cars than in the US because trains and buses abound.

Overall, the US has focused instead on building highways. Consequently, automobile ownership has monumentally grown since the early twentieth century. This has also raised automobile emissions into the atmosphere, posing an additional environmental hazard.

While many cities built extensive subway and public bus systems, we are still indeed an automobile-loving nation. However, people living in the suburbs and rural geographic areas have to depend significantly on automobile transportation to perform daily activities.

For elderly people across the US, who may no longer be able to drive, this can create tremendous difficulty in performing such essential activities as grocery shopping or seeing a doctor.

The existing US passenger railroad (*Amtrak*) has long been under-funded since fewer and fewer people ride it daily. Tracks in many areas are in such disrepair that no train can safely ride on them.

A recent article noted that *Amtrak (*as of May 2020*)* needs a $1.5 billion bailout to continue functioning.[46] We certainly are not England in terms of our valuation of railways!

How the Disparity in Reliable Transportation Affects the Health of People of Color

It is harder for low-income African American, Latinx, and Native American people to receive a car loan to purchase a new vehicle. Even when qualifying for a loan, low-income people tend to be offered a higher re-payment interest rate. Therefore, the overall cost of that new car is frequently more than for someone in a higher-income bracket.

Meanwhile, low-income people of color most often purchase used cars if they can afford a car in the first place. An unreliable vehicle can result in a person being late for work, which can result in losing their job.

Consequently, it can lead to defaulting on the automobile loan, the car being repossessed, and the credit score for acquiring a future car loan destroyed.

For a middle-class person of color, automobile loans can be more difficult to acquire than for a middle-class white person.

In 2013, the US Consumer Financial Protection Agency reasserted that discrimination in auto-lending is illegal. However, under the leadership of Mitch McConnell, Congress in 2018 reversed that guidance, paving the way for the resumption of widespread discriminatory practices in enabling auto loans.[47]

Understanding the Link Between Transportation and US Healthcare System Changes

For the past twenty years, a shift toward value-based payments has occurred in the health insurance landscape.

Prior to the mid-2000s, most hospitals and physicians were paid with a Fee-for-Service (FFS) model. Under an FFS model, hospitals and physicians were paid for each individual service they provided.

This payment system encouraged providing more tests and services to patients than they needed as a way to accrue more dollars from insurers, whether public or private.

In contrast, a value-based payment model reimburses hospitals and physicians based on patient care outcomes. Therefore, this model provides an incentive to be as cost-effective as possible while also providing excellent medical care (since high-quality delivered at low-cost results in a prodigious payment rate by insurers).

The US Centers for Medicare and Medicaid Services (CMS) shifted to this value-based payment model as a way to reign in national healthcare spending (as embraced by the *Affordable Care Act* [*ACA*]), which promoted the creation of Patient-Centered Medical Homes (PCMH) that would act as a team to provide coordinated patient care.

For example, a PCMH could include a hospital, a primary care doctor, some specialist physicians, a physical therapist (and other therapists), a social worker, and nursing staff. For patients, a PCMH can mean coordinated care that enables a more holistic approach.

Subsequent to the CMS shift, private insurers have similarly shifted toward adopting a value-based payment model. However, one unexpected consequence has been that physicians in rural areas, who more often worked in "solo" practices than suburban and urban physicians, needed to form networks to provide a PCMH to their patients.

Basically, this was the impetus for the development (and rapid expansion) of Accountable Care Organizations (ACO). These are large privately-owned hospitals and small healthcare practices that offer PCMHs, enabling a more costly payment rate, in turn, generating greater revenue for the ACO.

As the ACOs gobbled up small rural hospitals and solo practices, their locations were consolidated such that some rural areas no longer have a hospital within 100 miles.

The ACO also provided additional resources to rural hospitals and medical providers to offset the changing healthcare system landscape. Still, ACOs have continued to find ways to create competition for community hospitals resulting in the closure of many of them.

Regardless of whether the shift to value-based payments led to this problematic situation, the acceptance of nationwide healthcare as a business providing revenues to health insurers is the underlying cause of this problem.

Think about it. Chain department stores put many small clothing stores out of business. Therefore, it should be no surprise to anyone that ACOs are doing the same thing to small-sized hospitals and healthcare practices.

For rural residents, a trip to a hospital Emergency Department (ED) or physician's office can mean a car trip of sixty miles or more. This can make acquiring healthcare even more difficult for an African American, Latinx, or Native American individual living in a rural area, especially someone age sixty-five and older.

For rural residents, a trip to a hospital Emergency Department (ED) or physician's office can mean a car trip of sixty miles or more. This can make acquiring healthcare even more difficult for an African American, Latinx, or Native American individual living in a rural area, especially someone age sixty-five and older.

Urban geographic areas are the hub of teaching hospitals, so people with rare disorders are most expected to be referred by their primary care physician (PCP) to a specialist physician practicing in the nearest urban area.

However, lack of transportation can make the trip impossible, thereby contributing to a worsened health outcome.

Enough said about inequities in transportation access. You get the picture.

CHAPTER 5

Δ

FOOD AND NUTRITION

The most critical health-impacting factor is the quality of nutrition and food consumed. This is especially the case for infants and children, as nutritional deficiencies can lead to health disorders.

Because children's brains and bodies are still developing, a nutrient-related deficiency can lead to an escalated risk for many ailments in adulthood. In addition, they are a potential contributing factor to the infant mortality (death before the first birthday) disparities between Black and white babies.

Black babies have almost twice the risk of infant mortality when paralleled with children of white mothers. Not to mention the capacity for fostering permanent damage such as a weakened immune system.

According to a research article titled "Diet-Related Disparities: Understanding the Problem and Accelerating the Solution," Black and Brown people in the US tend to have inadequate nutrient profiles and dietary behaviors.[48]

One in every nine people in the US struggles with hunger. In 2017, at least forty million people in the US were food-insecure.[49] When children are hungry, they are far less able to concentrate in school.

Since 2016, federal food programs have been curtailed or defunded. The US African American population is twice as likely to face hunger as the white population, and eight of the ten counties with the largest food-insecurity rates in the US are at least 60% African American.[50]

People living in impoverished urban neighborhoods, particularly African American and Latinx individuals, can find it challenging to find any fresh produce to purchase. Additionally, people living in poverty are more expected to consume a high-carbohydrate diet since carbohydrates are more filling.

Correspondingly, low-income people working a full-time job (or all too often more than one job) can find it faster to prepare quick-cooking meals from packaged food items for their families rather than utilize more nutritious ingredients requiring more preparation and cooking time. Protein-rich foods also tend to cost more than high-carbohydrate food items.

Every vitamin and mineral has a Recommended Daily Allowance (RDA), and eating a balanced daily diet is the way to achieve this RDA by clinical nutritionists and other healthcare clinicians. Meanwhile, fast-food items that are available in stores located in Black and Brown neighborhoods tend to be abundant in carbohydrates and fats (but low in vitamins and minerals).

These include products widely marketed at children, so overworked, low-income parents who are exhausted may just give in to their children's request for an empty-calorie item to assuage their hunger. However, fast-food and empty-calorie items tend to have more calories, contributing to the ongoing obesity epidemic.

Some of the negative impacts of food insecurity are described in an article in 2018 in *Family and Community Medicine* as the following: higher rates of diabetes and hypertension, self-reported fair or ill health, maternal depression, and behavioral problems/developmental delays in early life.

This article also concluded that structural racism is the primary basis for this disparity between whites and people of color in the US.[51]

The Problem of Lost Nutritional Value in Foods Sold in Supermarkets

Most people in the western world purchase food rather than grow (or raise) what is eaten. This is in contrast to previous centuries when people mainly lived on farms or near their food sources.

In the US, much of our fresh produce is raised in California or Mexico and then transported to other areas of the country by truck and airplane.

The nutrient value of produce decreases during the time that it is being transported to processing and packaging centers. On average, once it makes it to supermarkets, it has been approximately seven to ten hours from farm to grocery.

Meanwhile, the meat industry in the US injects cows, pigs, and poultry with antibiotics to decrease their likelihood of mortality from bacterial infections and thereby preserve their animals for meat production. This contributes to the increase in antibiotic-resistant bacterial infections in humans since our bodies absorb these extra antibiotics.

In rural communities, especially in the Midwest and South, people are traveling farther to buy food due to chain supermarkets putting small (locally owned) supermarkets out of business.

In urban areas, impoverished neighborhoods are subjected to these chain grocery stores charging loftier prices (partially due to investing in more surveillance equipment to catch shoplifters and burglars and then passing that cost on to consumers). The only other option is small convenience stores, which tend to stock mostly pre-packaged, empty-calorie food items and no fresh produce.

"Food Deserts" and Public Health Responses

"We have food deserts in our cities. We know that the distance you live from a supplier of fresh produce is one of the best predictors of your health. And in the inner city, people don't have grocery stores. So, we have to find a way of getting supermarkets and farmers markets into the inner city." — US author Michael Pollan [52]

Impoverished communities that lack access to fresh and healthy foods are considered "food deserts" by public health professionals.

According to study findings published in the *Journal of the American Heart Association* (*JAHA*) in 2019, living in a food desert was associated with a heightened risk for cardiovascular disorders and an elevated resultant risk of death. [53]

One public health response in some cities has been supporting the creation of community gardens so that residents can grow fresh produce for their own consumption.

Obesity and Diabetes—Disparity in Prevalence Rates

Impoverished people are more likely to consume high-carbohydrate meals due to their lower cost, contributing to obesity. Meanwhile, empty-calorie items, especially appealing to children, most often have high sugar content. Once children get used to consuming a lot of sugar, it is harder for them to stop having that much sugar in their daily diet as adolescents and adults.

African American women have the largest obesity rates of any ethnic group in the United States. African Americans in 2018 were also 20% less likely to engage in daily physical exercise than non-Hispanic whites (per the US Office of Minority Health).[54]

African American adolescents also have higher obesity rates than white adolescents and particularly African American girls.[55]

Since obesity is strongly connected to the development of diabetes (Type 2), the disparity in the obesity rate requires attention to change this reality.

Cultural factors also contribute to the advanced obesity rates in African American and Latinx people. Many preferred (special) food items are high in either (or both) carbohydrate and sugar content. However, socioeconomic factors are the primary drivers underpinning the disparity in obesity and diabetes prevalence rates.

Meanwhile, obesity affects 40% of Native Americans (18% have diabetes). Moreover, Native Americans have the greatest risk of diabetes (both Type 1 [formerly termed *juvenile diabetes*] and Type 2) compared to all other ethnic groups in the US.[56]

Diabetes is one of the leading causes of kidney failure, and it is also associated with an increased risk for heart disease, retinopathy (leading to blindness), and premature death.

Diabetics also often suffer *diabetic neuropathy* (a type of nerve pain), which can be very debilitating and prevent remaining in the workforce. Therefore, changing dietary habits is crucial to avoid the development of Type 2 diabetes.

Poor Nutrition in Pregnancy — The Ramifications

Pregnant women living in poverty are far more likely to have nutritional deficiencies than women who are not impoverished. However, pregnant women under the age of twenty are also less likely to eat a nutritious diet and seek prenatal care.

This leads to a higher chance of developing pregnancy complications *and* giving birth to premature babies with concomitant lower-than-normal birthweight.

Low birthweight in the newborn is associated with furthered risk for infant mortality, underdeveloped organs, weak resistance to infection, and developmental delays that can appear as early as infancy.

Besides inadequate nutrition during pregnancy, three health disorders in pregnant women linked to low birthweight babies are diabetes, high blood pressure, and kidney disease.[57]

Meanwhile, pregnant women with poor nutritional status have an advanced risk of a complication called *eclampsia,* which can be life-threatening for both the pregnant woman and the fetus. Since many pregnant women do not get 100% of the RDA of vitamins and minerals recommended during pregnancy, taking vitamin supplements is often recommended at a prenatal healthcare visit.

Pregnant women need substantially more Folic Acid (a B-vitamin) than non-pregnant women, and the Centers for Disease Control (CDC) recommends that pregnant women take daily 400 mcg of Folic Acid in vitamin form in addition to consuming food with Folate (the naturally occurring form of Folic Acid) to avoid birth defects associated with low-Folate during pregnancy (*e.g., spina bifida* which is featured by lower extremity paralysis).[58]

Consider the following case and point. For a young, impoverished, pregnant woman with low educational attainment, the cost of Folic Acid in pill form may be unaffordable. Additionally, a lack of education may make understanding the need to take Folic Acid difficult.

Therefore, the woman might be unable to comply with her gynecologist's preventive health recommendation to take daily vitamin pills.

This is precisely the situation faced by many young Mexican American pregnant women. Now consider President Trump's executive order ("public charge rule") banning legal immigrants from applying for citizenship who already receive public benefits (such as Medicaid).[59]

That executive order, first proposed as a final rule in 2018, was enabled to go into effect by the Supreme Court on February 24, 2020.[60]

For a pregnant woman in this circumstance, her health and the health of her baby are both likely to needlessly suffer permanent damage.

Homelessness disproportionately affects people of color and eating healthy while homeless is nearly impossible.

Meanwhile, no one should have to choose whether to purchase needed food or prescription medication, but too many people living in poverty in the US are forced to make that choice. A significant number of them are also disabled or over age sixty-five with no way to return to employment.

Imagine how your life would have been different if you were or were not afforded certain opportunities. If you had or had not been set up for success by receiving the proper prenatal care.

There are many other social determinants of health, but these five are the most studied and documented by public health researchers. Therefore, these were selected for inclusion in this book. They were also important to cover because they are life-changing drivers on one's quality and, yes, quality of life.

Imagine how your life would have been different if you were or were not afforded certain opportunities. If you had or had not been set up for success by receiving the proper prenatal care.

Yes, one small influencer can and has made a world of difference, and as you read this book, I want you to wear a lens of reflection that stimulates a deep sense of awareness that energizes you to take action.

PART I

QUESTIONS TO PROMOTE YOUR THOUGHTS, KNOWLEDGE, AND SELF-AWARENESS

1.   Have you been affected by any of the five social determinants of health described in Part I? If so, how did these social determinants impact your health and/or access to healthcare?

_____

_____

_____

_____

_____

2.   Have any of your family members or friends been affected by the five social determinants of health described in Part I? If so, how did these social determinants impact their health and/or access to healthcare?

_____

_____

_____

_____

_____

3.   Have you ever felt that something in your housing situation was not healthy or safe for you? If so, what about your housing situation made you feel this way? How did you deal with your sense of a lack of healthfulness or safety in your housing situation?

_____

_____

_____

_____

_____

4.   Have you ever been homeless, known someone who was homeless, or met someone homeless? How did you feel about your homelessness or the homelessness of someone else, and what did you do about it?

_____

_____

_____

_____

5.   Have you ever felt that you (or someone you know) was not treated fairly in school or an educational setting? If so, why?

_____

_____

_____

_____

6.   Have you ever felt that you (or someone you know) were the victim of discrimination in employment? If so, why?

_____

_____

_____

_____

_____

7.   How do you travel to your healthcare appointments, and is this mode of transportation satisfactory for your needs?

_____

_____

_____

_____

_____

8.   Are you satisfied with your weight, or do you feel too heavy or too thin? If so, have you attempted recently to do anything to change your weight? What did you do to try to change your weight (if you have ever tried to lose or gain weight)?

_____

_____

_____

_____

_____

9. Do you eat at least one serving of fresh fruit and vegetables each week? If not, why not?

_____

_____

_____

_____

_____

10. Are you able to purchase fresh fruits and vegetables from your local grocery store (or some other store near your home or work) each week? If not, why not?

_____

_____

_____

_____

_____

OTHER FACTORS CONTRIBUTING TO HEALTH DISPARITIES IN THE US

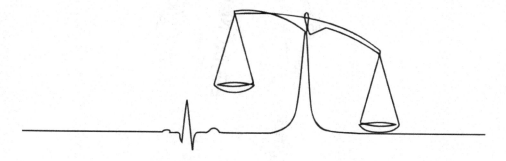

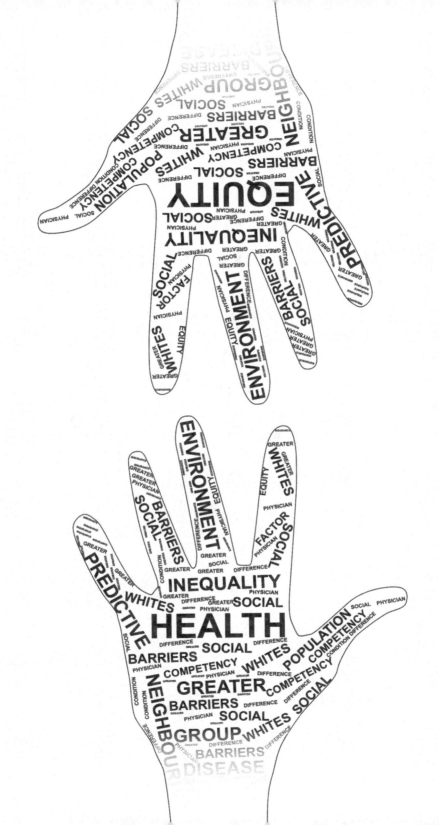

CHAPTER 6

Δ

HISTORICAL INAPPROPRIATE MEDICAL CARE OF BLACK AND BROWN PEOPLE

busive medical treatment of African American, Latinx, and Native American people has a very long history. You may be familiar with the forty-year Tuskegee Experiment conducted by the US Public Health Service, in which unsuspecting African American male volunteers with syphilis were promised treatment.

Instead, half were given medication, and half were given a placebo (a drug capsule with nothing in it) to compare the outcomes over time. The recipients were not told that they had never received the medication that could have cured them until they had reached the end-of-life stage of disease progression.[61]

In *The Immortal Life of Henrietta Lacks*,[62] American science writer and New York Times bestselling author, Rebecca Skloot, describes how a young, African American woman (whose story is core to this investigative exposé) developed terrible pain from uterine cancer.

She was initially misdiagnosed by a white doctor who, without examining her, assumed the cause of her pain was psychological. Around a year later, she was treated with radium inserted into her (which is carcinogenic) and died.

Meanwhile, without her knowledge or that of her family members, her cancer cells were kept for research purposes and sold worldwide to clinical research centers studying uterine cancer treatments.

Then there were the 1993 New York State Psychiatric Institute (NYSPI) experiments that took place over three years. In one of the experiments, thirty-four New York City boys between the ages of six and ten, all of whom were Black and Hispanic, were given fenfluramine.

This is an appetite suppressant that was banned in 1997 due to safety concerns. These boys' names were taken through the Board of Corrections. They were the younger siblings of men already in the criminal justice system. These boys were given this drug intravenously to test the theory that criminal behavior could be predicted by brain chemical levels.

Patient advocacy groups argued that these young boys were used in experiments without any hope of medical benefit despite being exposed to significant risk. *The New York Times* ran this story in April of 1998.

Forced Sterilization as a Racist Strategy for Population Control

Forced sterilization has been perpetrated on women of color in various periods throughout US history and is primarily a means to curb the population growth of groups of people considered "less desirable."

Embraced by President Woodrow Wilson, it was the Eugenics Movement's core belief in white supremacy that underpinned the first US law allowing forced sterilization in 1904.[63] It was this same Eugenics Movement that formed the intellectual basis for Hitler's genocide against Jews.

In the 1960s, one-third of all Puerto Rican women living in Puerto Rico or on the US mainland were forcibly sterilized.[64] However, one of the first legal cases that generated public outrage in the US against forced sterilization occurred a decade later.

Two African American girls aged twelve and fourteen (the Relf sisters in 1973) were sterilized against their will. Their mother had provided consent under the false premise by a health center that the girls would be given birth control.

The Southern Poverty Law Center filed a federal case that year (*Relf v. Weinberger*) on their behalf, but the case was dismissed.[65]

Meanwhile, a mass sterilization campaign of Native American women was conducted between 1960 and 1980 as implemented by the US Indian Health Services.[66]

Around 70,000 recorded female "sterilizations-without-consent" occurred in the US during these two decades.[67]

Under President Nixon's policy directive, Medicaid funding in the 1970s for sterilization was dramatically amplified (targeted at Black and Brown women living in poverty). In 1981, the last legally allowed forced sterilization occurred in Oregon.[68]

It is no wonder that so many African American, Latinx, Asian American, and Native American women feel mistrustful of the healthcare system.

Medical Providers' Disrespect of African Americans

There are good reasons to be reluctant to visit a white doctor if you are African American. Too many African American patients' complaints of pain are not taken seriously. Perhaps you have had this experience yourself.

Per an article in 2016 published in the *Proceedings of the National Academy of Sciences*, African Americans are systematically undertreated for pain relative to white Americans.[69]

Likewise, the Association of American Medical Colleges (AAMC) in 2020 reported, "Half of white medical trainees believe such myths as black people have thicker skin or less sensitive nerve endings than white people."

This AAMC webpage also described findings of a research study in 2016 that revealed 40% of the surveyed first and second-year white medical students held stereotype-based (false) views pertaining to African American bodies.[70]

While not all white physicians are this ignorant, it is yet another potential hurdle for any African American in need of ongoing medical care (especially in rural and suburban areas where most of the local physicians have rarely cared for an African American patient).

Meanwhile, most active physicians in the US are white (56.2%), while only 2.6% of the nation's doctors in 2019 and 7.3% of students enrolled in medical school in 2020 identified as Black or African American.

This is a 13% lag in the overall population.[71] In 2019, only 3.8% of doctors identified as Hispanic, Latino, or of Spanish origin.

What Does Disrespect Look Like?

The following happened to a woman that I will call "Janet" (fictional name), a low-income, African American woman in her thirties with a mild developmental disability.

After experiencing stabbing chest pains and feeling weak when standing, she had a friend drive her to a hospital Emergency Department (ED) to seek medical care, where she was quickly triaged and diagnosed with a heart attack. Afterward, surgery was performed on Janet to place heart stents. So far, so good.

However, three days later, Janet was discharged home. Shortly before discharge, a prescription was "called in" by her physician to a local pharmacy for a blood-thinner to reduce the likelihood that Janet would develop a blood clot and have a second heart attack.

That same afternoon, Janet was driven by a neighbor to the pharmacy to pick up her prescription, only to discover that Medicaid would not cover the cost. Since Janet could not afford to pay for this expensive medication herself, she did not obtain it.

Only six days after her discharge from the hospital, Janet phoned her sister, who works in the medical field. She told her sister that she was again having a hard time breathing and generally felt horrible. Her sister then phoned Janet's Primary Care Physician (PCP), who prescribed a Medicaid-covered medication to substitute for the hospital-prescribed drug.

Despite filling this prescription, six days after her original discharge from the hospital, this woman's breathing, and other symptoms had *increased* rather than *decreased*. Her sister (who could not leave work early) phoned a cousin to take Janet back to the emergency room, although she planned to follow up at the emergency department after her shift had ended.

When her sister arrived at the ED two hours later, Janet was still sitting in the lobby. Janet told her sister that the ED's registration clerk instructed her to wait. Outraged, her sister stressed to the registration clerk the need for immediate attention.

Janet received attention from a physician within ten minutes and subsequently was rushed into emergency surgery (as constriction of the heart stents had occurred). Although Janet survived, she was left with *preventable* but permanent heart damage.

Would this have happened to someone in a different socioeconomic class, race, or level of education? Would a different outcome have occurred if Janet were covered by some other insurance instead of Medicaid?

Would Janet have waited so long if she was given adequate information at her first appointment regarding the serious nature of her condition? These are all questions for you to consider in reflecting on what happened to Janet after her health crisis.

My primary point in beginning this section with this story is to foster your awareness that a wide range of factors must be considered in examining "what disrespect looks like!"

Perhaps it will not surprise you that research has shown that African Americans have historically waited longer in a hospital Emergency Department to receive care than white patients.[72]

Anyone who has been disrespected by a healthcare clinician or staff member is well aware of how it *feels*, but all too often, disrespect based on racism is *covert*, which means it is not blatant (or *overt*) enough to file any official discrimination complaint.

Body language (suggesting disbelief or disinterest), lack of eye contact, and rushing through a medical examination and/or explanation are just a few examples of how covert racism is all too often displayed.

Although more subtle than saying "you are not worthy of my time," the message comes across loud and clear to a person on the receiving end. I've been there, and it does not feel good!

However, some progress has been made, and the *Black Lives Matter* movement is focusing far more attention on *covert* racism than before this movement existed.

Meanwhile, over the past decade, medical schools have been increasingly including "cultural competence" as a required course for their students to complete their training and then begin a medical resident training period (residency) in their chosen specialty.

Prominent medical centers are trending toward requiring the attendance of clinicians at periodic "cultural competence" workshops. Likewise, the necessary annual Continuing Education Units (CEUs) for physicians, nurses, and allied health professionals can more often be partially acquired through attending an in-person or online course in "cultural competence."

Perpetual experiences of disrespect can lead to an overall distrust of healthcare providers. An article in the *American Journal of Community Psychology* stated, "Mistrust of healthcare organizations and health professionals has been associated with less care satisfaction, treatment adherence, and utilization of healthcare services."[73]

Unfortunately, this article, which focuses on the healthcare provider experiences of African American males, did not discuss the problem of physician disrespect for the patient as contributing in any way to this outcome.

An analysis of study findings (published in 2019 in *PLoS One*) showed that 40% of the 1,543 study participants reported at least one type of perceived discrimination in a medical setting; this discrimination was perceived across health settings from a variety of healthcare providers and staff.[74]

Furthermore, these findings revealed that perceived discrimination in medical settings was associated with reporting not having enough time with the physician and not being enabled to participate in decision-making as much as desired.

In answer to a survey question about the quality of healthcare service received, 40% of African American respondents (who felt the service quality was poor) linked this to a perception of a discriminatory healthcare experience.

Mexican Americans who participated in this study were less likely to associate a perception of bad service quality with race-based discrimination, and, no surprise, whites were less likely to report discrimination than any of the three groups of study participants of color.[75]

Three identified ways that physicians and providers have demonstrated prejudice against African American patients have been disinterest in their health concerns, perceived lack of attention, and self-reported difference in interpersonal interactions between healthcare providers and themselves as compared to the providers' patients who were not from underrepresented populations (*Journal of Black Studies*).[76]

A sad reality is that repeated race-based discriminatory experiences with healthcare providers and facilities can facilitate distrust in all medical professionals. You can think of it as akin to a Post-Traumatic Stress Disorder (PTSD) response, in that a sound or facial expression can trigger flashbacks and associations even when the distressing experience at present is not being repeated.

However, *not* receiving medical care when needed is harmful to overall health, so avoiding seeking healthcare is not a good approach to coping with a fear of encountering a racist healthcare provider.

If you are African American and seeking a new Primary Care Physician (PCP), specialist, or surgeon, interviewing that healthcare provider may enable you to ascertain if that physician has ignorant beliefs. As a matter of fact, regardless of race, interview *all* new physicians to ensure it is a good fit.

Do not just entrust your care to anyone without doing your homework. Take ownership and become an empowered and engaged member of your healthcare journey.

Do not just entrust your care to anyone without doing your homework. Take ownership and become an empowered and engaged member of your healthcare journey.

While you may not be able to tell through one conversation, meeting that person before entrusting your healthcare to his/her judgment is a reasonable approach.

Health insurance that requires utilization of only "in-network" physicians may limit your options, but most physicians and nurse practitioners will allow a brief interview with a prospective patient if requested.

Disrespect Aimed at Physicians of Color

The disrespect problem is not one only underwent by Black and Brown patients. It is also one experienced by African American and other minority physicians. Black and Brown medical students and physicians are often assaulted by microaggressions perpetrated by their superiors and colleagues.

This can include disparaging remarks, lack of access to mentors, and inequities in career advancement potential, pay, and benefits.

While these are not the most volatile acts of racism, they build into a culture that is not conducive to a healthy work environment. Just so it lets people know that even if they don't think those are that bad, they do create monumental difficulties.

According to "Racism as Experienced by Physicians of Color in the Healthcare Setting" by *Family Medicine*, racism perpetrated by *patients* in the form of refusal to allow care by that physician for race-based reasons was reported by 23% of studied physicians.

This article also noted that physicians reported they were more likely to face racism from their colleagues than their patients.[77]

Consequently, physician dissatisfaction among physicians of color is heightened. This does not always occur at a level in accordance with the race-based disrespect endured (as burnout is most prevalent among white physicians[78]).

Indeed, findings of a study published in *Health Equity* suggested that Black and Brown physician participants self-reported symptoms related to burnout at lower rates than white physicians.

This may be due to a higher degree of coping skills/resilience, as a consequence of having to overcome more barriers to achieving a career as a physician *in tandem* with a sense of obligation of contributing to their communities.[79]

On the other hand, physicians are also patients, and prolonged stress can contribute to chronic health disorders common in middle age. Not suitable for physician health and well-being!

Another problematic issue is the population running healthcare facilities such as hospitals, clinical trials centers, pharmaceutical companies, and nonprofit health centers. Among US hospitals, only 14% of Board Members and 9% of CEOs are people of color.[80]

Additionally, the senior leadership teams do not represent the population for which their health care organization was established to serve. There is a lack of diversity above, and the gap is significant.

Since administrative leadership impacts hospital policies, including requirements for a baseline of cultural competence among its employees, this disparity also needs to change.

Therefore, raised recruitment nationwide of Black and Brown medical professionals in all areas of the healthcare system needs to occur. This will help reduce the scope of the microaggressions experienced by Black and Brown medical providers and patients alike.

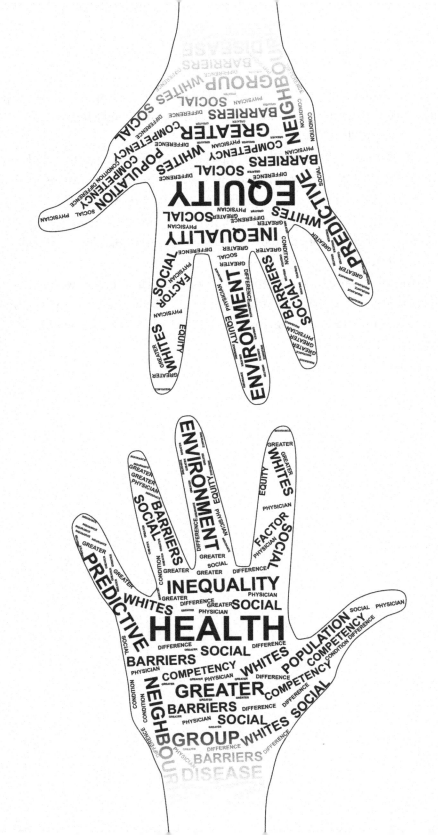

CHAPTER 7

Δ

BIAS AMONG HEALTHCARE PROVIDERS AND IN MEDICAL/NURSING SCHOOL TRAINING

The previous chapter discussed race-based bias in healthcare settings affecting patients and introduced bias aimed at physicians. However, the prejudice encountered by patients and healthcare providers of color is also based on assumptions about Black and Brown socioeconomic status.

Before we move further into the discussion, let me talk about explicit versus implicit. I do not believe that most physicians wake up, go to their offices, and set out to act explicitly racist to their patients. However, implicit racism all too often rears its ugly head, regardless of intent to do so.

Implicit racism and unconscious/implicit prejudice are involuntarily triggered and can unintentionally occur (and *does* occur) during our daily interactions. Physicians are no exception, regardless of their race.

For example, an African American female, who is a hypertensive diabetic, presents for a medical visit. Her physician tells her that she needs to lose weight for her hypertension to decrease.

He is cognitive of the fact that she cannot afford a gym membership. Therefore, this physician gives her a treatment plan that includes walking thirty to forty-five minutes for three days every week somewhere close to where she lives. Unfortunately, she lives in a not-so-safe neighborhood, with no sidewalks, parks , or greenspaces within reasonable walking distance.

This physician's implicit bias grew out of the reality that everyone this physician knows resides in safe neighborhoods with sidewalks and lots of green space.

Therefore, this physician makes the assumption that the same is true for everyone. In other words, it is not in this physician's worldview to recognize that some people do not have this physician's lifestyle and privileges.

Equity is not a stand-alone initiative. It should be woven into the fabric of every endeavor you embark upon and every interaction with every patient. No decision should be made without applying the equity lens.

In other words, due to hidden cognitive bias, this physician not only cannot conceive of life for someone without similar privileges but has never *tried* to conceive of life for someone without access to those privileges!

Equity is not a stand-alone initiative. It should be woven into the fabric of *every* endeavor you embark upon and *every* interaction with *every* patient. No decision should be made without applying the equity lens.

Health outcomes are directly connected to where a person lives, works, worships and plays. In 2016, the sixteenth Surgeon General, David Satcher, observed that 84,000 members of the minority community in the US die each year due to disparities in care.

If you are interested in the realm of unconscious bias, the Harvard University-designed *Implicit Association Test* (*IAT*) is a tool designed to enable us to recognize and identify our implicit biases.

The purpose of this online test is to measure implicit attitudes and beliefs that we are unwilling (or unable) to detect, report, and become intentional about in terms of changing these attitudes/beliefs. This test is free; its results are described as confidential, and it can be accessed at http://implicit.harvard.edu/implicit.[81]

According to the Institute of Medicine's book, *Unequal Treatment: Confronting Racial and Ethnic Disparities in Health Care,* African American and Latinx patients, in general, are more disposed to be assumed impoverished and, therefore, with less health insurance coverage by healthcare providers upon the first encounter.[82]

This stereotyping of the socioeconomic class of Black and Brown individuals

by healthcare professionals in a medical setting can lead to inequities in scheduling appointments and overall treatment.

Allow me to digress for a moment and share with you another personal story.
In 2013 I injured my hand late in the evening and needed to visit the ED for
stitches. The physician assistant sutured me up, and upon discharge, the physician
told me to come back in three days to have my sutures removed.

As a healthcare professional, my first thought was: that is not the appropriate
recommendation for suture removal. The visit should be with my PCP. But wait,
let me backup and provide you with a more detailed account of what actually
occurred

The ED physician made minimal eye contact with me. On two separate occa-
sions during this visit, I informed him that I could not move my pinky finger, and
both times I was dismissed. He delegated a physician assistant (PA) to suture my
hand. Within five minutes, he entered the room and scolded the PA.

"What is taking you so long? You're not stitching a limb back on. Hurry up!"
he barked.

The PA nervously continued the process as I assured him that he was
doing fine and to not be shaken. The doctor then came back into the room
about ten minutes later and without asking me any questions or providing any
discharge instructions, told me to follow up in five to seven days to have my
sutures removed.

Based on how I was treated by him throughout this visit, I knew he assumed
I was uninsured. How about referring me to the hand surgeon that I obviously
needed?

However, I politely informed him that suture removal was not appropriate
utilization of the ED and that I would be following up with my PCP. These
bigoted assumptions not only impact the patient but the overall system. Totally
unacceptable!

One reason this class-based inequity in scheduling and treatment can occur
is that outpatient clinicians, whether general practitioners or specialists, may need
to limit their acceptance of new patients on Medicaid and/or reduce the likeli-

hood of failure to receive payment to maximize their practice's revenues to maintain financial viability.

Physicians in outpatient and various allied health practices can also assume that a new Black or Brown patient will require more attention from their staff due to a stereotype-based expectation of there being more health disorders in patients of color.

Meanwhile, physicians, nurses, and allied healthcare professionals are often assumed to be less competent if African American, Latinx, or Asian by white healthcare professionals and other workplace staff. It is not unusual for African American physicians to be confused as custodians or aides by employees and patients in a healthcare environment. Even by Black and Brown employees and patients!

Time for another quick story, this time not personal, but nevertheless another real-life example. An African American male nurse had been assigned to a middle-aged white male for his shift.

He introduced himself and started his work. Each time he entered the room during his shift, the man called him Tobi. Although his name did begin with the letter T, it was not remotely close to Tobi. Despite being corrected each time, he refused to call him by his correct name.

Okay, let's pause. Kunta Kinte is a character in the 1976 novel *Roots* by author Alex Haley. He was sold into slavery and renamed Tobi. He was not willing to acknowledge this name and was beaten into submission. Imagine how this young man, this registered nurse, this African American medical professional, felt.

The Nursing and Allied Healthcare Workforce

According to a national survey of the nursing workforce, only 19% of all Registered Nurses (RNs) are people of color. Of these RNs, 6% were African American (which is below the 13% of African Americans in the US population). Only 5% were Latino/Hispanic, and less than 1% were Native American. Meanwhile, nearly 7% were Asian, and 81% were white.

The gender breakdown for all nurses was 93% female and 7% male, but this breakdown was 92% female and 8% male among African Americans.[83]

The degree most attained for the first nursing license was a two-year associate's degree (38%), followed by a four-year baccalaureate degree (36%). However, among actively practicing African American RNs, the nursing degree first attained was most often a B.S. degree (50%) followed by an A.S. degree (27.6%).

The increased pay and respect afforded by supervisors for nurses with B.S. degrees may be the driving force behind this preference since African Americans who are inclined to acquire acceptance into an RN program know they will face racism as an additional obstacle in any chosen healthcare occupation.

Therefore, attaining a higher-level nursing degree may feel like a deterrent against future race-based discrimination as career nurses.

Additionally, this national nursing survey revealed the following statistics. Among Licensed Practical Nurses (LPNs) and Licensed Vocational Nurses (LVNs), who only require a one-year degree, African Americans were three times more likely to be LPNs/LVNs than RNs.

Around 16% of all LPNs/LVNs in the US are African American. The corresponding Latino/Hispanic rates were substantially lower than for African Americans with LPN/LVNs (7.4%) and RNs (5.3%).

63% of RNs work in hospitals, and only 7% work in nursing homes.[84] However, African American nurses are disproportionately represented in nursing homes and as homecare nurses. By the same token, LPNs/LVNs are also more likely to work in nursing homes or homecare agencies.

The working conditions in nursing homes are notoriously terrible for nurses, with far fewer advancement opportunities than hospitals.

Nurses in nursing homes are also paid annually approximately $20,000 on average less than nurses in hospitals, and homecare nurses often are not hired as full-time employees with benefits. Homecare nurses are also generally expected to provide their own transportation to each patient's apartment or home and transport the needed supplies to treat their patients.

Since Black and Brown high school students are more predisposed to be steered toward a post-high school vocational program, it is no wonder that so many still choose to become an LPN/LVN despite this being a dead-end in today's nursing job market!

For those who choose to pursue a B.S. in Nursing, racist instructors, students, and patients can add a high degree of stress to an already stressful educational marathon toward launching a career.

In contrast to Black and Brown female medical students, nursing students of color are far more susceptible to experience sexual harassment by physicians and other staff members during their clinical learning experiences.

As if this was not dismal enough, studies have concluded 71% of *all* female nurses have been sexually harassed by patients;[85] female nurses of color are at an even more elevated risk of being sexually harassed in their workplace.

During the Covid-19 pandemic, nursing homes have been significantly impacted. Therefore, nurses of color working in nursing homes have been widely recognized as at heightened risk of contracting this coronavirus and, thereby, infecting their own family members. This is just one more inequity faced by Black and Brown nurses— on whom so many elderly Americans depend— in the healthcare workplace.

CHAPTER 8

Δ

BIG TOBACCO AND OPIOID MANUFACTURERS— IMPACT ON AFRICAN AMERICAN, LATINX, AND NATIVE AMERICAN PEOPLE

U S tobacco companies strategically marketed their products to African Americans in the 1950s and 1960s. Through this, they succeeded in appealing to a large proportion of African Americans (and other people of color) to purchase their products.

According to the Centers for Disease Control (CDC), "tobacco companies have historically placed sizable amounts of advertising in African American publications, exposing African Americans to more cigarette ads than Whites."[86]

The CDC also notes that large US tobacco companies have also aggressively marketed their products to African American youth in urban areas.

Next, in the late 1970s and 1980s, as anti-smoking campaigns were beginning to decrease cigarette purchases by white people in the US, tobacco companies began using US Census Bureau data to track demographic trends to target marketing initiatives at the Latino/Hispanic market.[87]

According to the American Lung Association, smoking rates are as follows: Native Americans/Alaska Natives (22%), African Americans (16.8%), Latinos/ Hispanics (10%), Asian Americans (7%), and non-Hispanic whites (16.6%).[88]

In the Latinx community, smoking prevalence varies by origin. Puerto Ricans have the largest smoking rates in the US, while Dominicans have the lowest.[89]

The cost of cigarettes has risen dramatically since the 1960s, partly due to state-imposed taxes to promote anti-smoking public health measures. Despite being one of the most addictive substances, smokers (especially those who began smoking in adolescence or younger) continue to purchase cigarettes despite the raised expense. Never mind the cost to health.

As noted in the *Journal of Environment and Health Sciences*, tobacco smoke contains more than 7,000 chemicals, including hundreds that are toxic and about seventy that can cause cancer.[90]

Smoking has been correlated to an enhanced risk of nearly every chronic health disorder and premature death. Meanwhile, secondhand smoke is recognized as a significant risk factor for asthma in children.

For Black and Brown people already at risk for chronic disorders, smoking increases their chances. This is also true for e-cigarettes which include carcinogens, volatile organic compounds, and heavy metals.[91]

According to the *International Journal of Environmental Research and Public Health*, e-cigarettes are used less among African American smokers than both Latino/Hispanic or white smokers, with the hugest prevalence among white smokers.

One possible reason provided by this article is that e-cigarette use is often started to begin smoking cessation.[92]

Meanwhile, Native Americans have the loftiest tobacco-smoking rate in the US at 32% but tend to not utilize mass-produced cigarettes or other mass-produced tobacco products.[93]

People incarcerated in prisons in the US, of whom most are African American, often use cigarettes to barter with the guards and other prisoners for perks, so it should come as no surprise to public health professionals that they leave prison addicted to cigarettes.

Heart Disease and Smoking

Smokers have a two-to-four-fold increased risk of developing coronary artery disease (CAD) and a 70% higher risk of death from CAD than non-smokers.[94]

A chief reason is that smoking boosts plaque formation in the blood vessels, including the arteries leading to the heart. Due to the growing obesity rate in Black and Brown people, smoking can be a double jeopardy as a link to early death.

For many smokers, disability and lowered quality of life arrive first. Since African American and Latinx people are less likely to have jobs providing health insurance (and more likely to be covered by Medicaid or have no insurance coverage), living with heart disease can be even more difficult than for the white population.

Procuring Social Security benefits for permanent disability often takes at least twelve months of waiting, so those diagnosed with heart disease who can no longer work may sink into dire financial straits.

Consequently, they may forego follow up with a cardiologist after a first heart attack and withhold their heart medication, which is typically expensive. This is just another illustration of why quitting smoking is an extremely good decision for those who smoke—and particularly for Black and Brown people.

Disparities in Smoking Cessation Program Participation for People of Color

Insurance plans may cover participation in a smoking cessation program but with a required co-pay from the participant for each session.

The Affordable Care Act (ACA) does not require state Medicaid programs to cover individual, group, or telephone cessation counseling for non-pregnant, adult Medicaid enrollees (per the CDC website).[95]

Therefore, even though the ACA does mandate coverage of most preventive healthcare, participating in a smoking cessation program may be too expensive for a low-income person of color.

Indeed, all of the social determinants that lead to health and healthcare inequities are at play when it comes to Black or Brown smokers attempting to quit smoking, *thereby potentially improving future health and quality of life.*

The Opioid Pharmaceutical Industry and Its
Impact on the Health of People of Color

You may be aware of the legal victory by a myriad of state and municipal governments against Purdue Pharma in 2019 as the developer and manufacturer of *OxyContin*, the first prescription opioid medication.[96]

One reason for the legal ruling against Purdue Pharma was that this company falsely marketed opioids to physicians as non-addictive for patients suffering from chronic pain.[97]

Since Black and Brown males disproportionately hold manual labor jobs, back pain, joint injuries, and/or arthritis are often the consequence. This is also true for home health aides, housecleaners, and restaurant workers.

Obesity can also contribute to joint damage (especially in the hips and knees) over the years. Meanwhile, people afflicted with the painful Sickle Cell Anemia, a genetic disorder that predominately affects Africans and African Americans,[98] have often been prescribed opioids to control their pain.[99] Additionally, diabetics with severe neuropathy may be prescribed opioids for pain control.[100]

As already described in an earlier chapter, some physicians believe that Black and Brown people have an increased capacity over white people to "tough out the pain" and "be strong."

For this reason, these physicians elect not to prescribe the necessary pain medication. In addition, there is a lack of trust on the physicians' part that Black and Brown patients will improperly take their prescription, as well as an unfounded belief that Black and Brown patients will sell the medication on the street rather than use it themselves.[101]

The problem now is that people of color who justly need opioids for pain are often unable to fill a prescription.

The high-pressure marketing campaign by Purdue Pharma (as well as various other pharmaceutical companies) to physicians to prescribe oxycodone painkillers to anyone with pain (including a toothache) resulted in the opioid epidemic in the 2000s. Black and

Brown people were disproportionately impacted and became addicted to their prescribed medications.

The ramifications are still being felt today. Many people who became dependent on oxycodone turned to heroin when they could not legally obtain more oxycodone. Financial ruin, destroyed family relationships, and homelessness were all too-frequent consequences of an addiction that started with prescribed pain medication.

As previously stated, the problem now is that people of color who justly need opioids for pain are often unable to fill a prescription.

Due to racial bias, many physicians assume that Black and Brown people in severe pain will abuse opioids, so they are reluctant to prescribe them for pain relief even when needed.[102]

For example, knee replacement surgery patients are often prescribed a week of opioids due to the severe post-surgical pain; this enables them to participate in their physical therapy and thereby return to normal walking. Without opioid medication, the recuperation period can be longer *and* excruciating.

People undergoing gum graft surgeries in dentists' offices can also face severe pain. However, dentists are even more reluctant than physicians to prescribe opioid medications for their patients, and most are not willing to prescribe *any* opioids for any reason to patients for fear of state public health action against them.[103]

Meanwhile, the opioid epidemic in the US— while not increasing at its previous rate, due to the decreased availability of prescription opioids— still rages on in terms of its consequences.

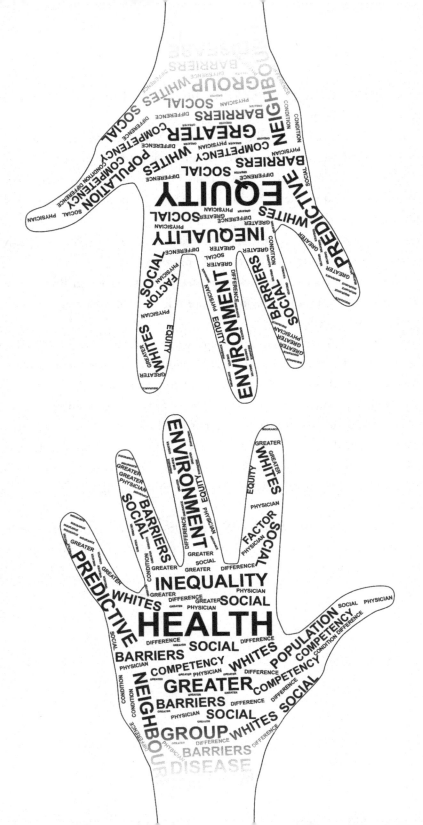

CHAPTER 9

Δ

MENTAL HEALTH AND SUBSTANCE ABUSE DISORDER AND ACCESS TO TREATMENT

One of the healthcare realms in which Black and Brown people fare the worst is mental health and substance abuse disorder treatment. Although one in five adults in the US suffer significant psychological distress, African American, Latinx, Asian, and Native American people are far less inclined to seek or receive mental health services than white people.[104]

Rates of mental illnesses in African Americans are similar to those of the general population. However, disparities exist regarding mental health care services.

Given the pervasive history of race-based discrimination in the US and boosted Black and Brown burden of chronic health disorders, is it any wonder that people of color in the US have a high degree of depression, anxiety, and PTSD?

Indeed, depression and anxiety may be the *same* reaction to the insanity of the abuse perpetrated against people of color.

It is vital to realize that the DMS (*Diagnostic and Statistical Manual of Mental Disorders*) of the American Psychiatric Association is the standard by which insurers (Medicare/Medicaid and private insurers) determine whether to cover the cost of a visit to a mental health counselor, psychologist, or psychiatrist.

Therefore, there needs to be a diagnosis reported from the DSM for the provider to get paid by the insurance company. Meanwhile, the DSM changes periodically to reflect current perceptions (*e.g.*, *Asperger's Syndrome* is now a subcategory of *Autism Spectrum Disorder*).

In terms of thinking about mental health disorders, this creates a limitation in that, not every person experiencing psychological distress actually fits neatly into a diagnosis described in the DSM. However, a diagnosis from the DSM still needs to be reported by the mental health therapist to be paid for each session with the client!

> *People of color are also disproportionately diagnosed with more disruptively labeled disorders, such as oppositional defiance disorder.*

Furthermore, DSM classifications affect everyone's perception of mental health disorders, and one consequence is the "medicalization" of human psychological distress, such that medications are often prescribed as a first-line approach rather than as a last resort approach.

People of color are also disproportionately diagnosed with more disruptively labeled disorders, such as oppositional defiance disorder (ODD) rather than attention deficit hyperactive disorder (ADHD). While these disorders share similar symptoms, the language behind them powers how people view those diagnosed.

Depression and Its Impact on People of Color

Clinical depression is a DSM classification that includes persistent feelings of depression. Around 7% of adults in the US are considered to have major depressive events that could progress to clinical depression—with depression prevalence among females of 8.7% and males of 5.3%.[105]

People of color are more susceptible to feel persistently depressed than white adults,[106] but only one in three African Americans who need mental health counseling seek and receive such services.[107]

Meanwhile, only one in ten Latinx people will seek an appointment with a mental health therapist.[108]

The following statistics from the US Office of Minority Health present the disparities in the experience of severe psychological distress in the past thirty days among adults eighteen years of age or older. The percentages were 3.6% (non-Hispanic-Black) and 3.7% (Non-Hispanic-White).

However, the rates were significantly higher among people living in poverty at 7.6% (non-Hispanic Black) and 12.1% (Non-Hispanic-White).[109]

Some research studies have even suggested that white people are less able to cope with life's setbacks/difficulties and become more depressed than Black and Brown people.[110]

Meanwhile, Black and Brown males are also less likely to seek or receive mental health services than females of color.[111]

It is well-recognized that depression exacerbates the risk of a suicide attempt.[112] However, even among depressed people who do not attempt suicide, prolonged depression can be harmful to their quality of life, interpersonal relationships, and overall health and well-being.

According to a research article in *Frontiers in Psychiatry*, clinical depression is the fourth-leading cause of disability and a prominent cause of non-fatal disease burden.

However, this article also suggests that African Americans have a lower lifetime rate of major depression than whites but also have reduced access to services and receive inferior services than whites.[113]

Anxiety Disorders and People of Color

Living with an anxiety disorder is not the same as feeling anxious. Instead, it is prolonged anxiety that is difficult to control, and more often than not, interferes with activities of daily living.

An article in the *Journal of Anxiety Disorders* specifies that panic disorder (PD), agoraphobia (AGO), social phobia (SAD), post-traumatic stress disorder (PTSD), and generalized anxiety disorder (GAD) are among the most prevalent psychiatric disorders in the US.[114]

Many people are diagnosed with both depression and anxiety. Among people living with a mental health disorder, this is one of the subgroups most liable to use alcohol to self-treat their mental health disorder.[115]

Obviously, this dependence upon alcohol can lead to alcoholism. The vicious cycle associated with this self-treatment is that alcohol depresses brain transmission of Serotonin (a neurotransmitter that boosts mood), so consuming alcohol actually worsens symptoms of clinical depression and anxiety.

According to the Anxiety and Depression Association of America, only 33% of those suffering from an anxiety disorder receive treatment.[116]

Therefore, it can be assumed based on wide recognition of the reduced acquisition of mental health services by people of color compared to white people that Black and Brown people with anxiety disorders receive even less treatment.

On the other hand, Black and Brown people are more likely to be treated solely with medication for mental health disorders than a combination of therapy and medication.[117]

Bipolar Disorder and People of Color

This severe and persistent mental illness (SPMI) is often featured by swings from depression to euphoria (although some people living with this disorder primarily suffer prolonged episodes of depression). A biological basis is generally believed to be the cause, and medication is typically prescribed to control symptoms.

While it is considered to affect people of color and white people equally, Black and Brown patients are less likely to receive a timely diagnosis and treatment than white patients.[118]

People afflicted with bipolar disorder are also more prone to abuse alcohol and drugs than people without this disorder and to display symptoms when not on symptom-controlling medication.

For people of color with untreated bipolar disorder, intimate relationships can become fractured, jobs can be lost, and this lack of stability may lead to incarceration.

This possible incarceration is also more likely to happen to them than the white population living with bipolar disorder since treatment in people of color is more often delayed until symptoms are severe.

Schizophrenia and People of Color

This SPMI is featured by auditory and visual hallucinations, as well as delusions. In contrast to bipolar disorder, which is classified as a mood disorder, schizophrenia is a disorder of thought processes.

Paranoid schizophrenia is typically featured by the belief that a conspiracy against the individual is occurring, resulting in persecution, along with the usual schizophrenia symptoms. Although it affects less than 1% of the population, schizophrenia is the most disabling major mental health disorder.[119]

It also is the psychiatric disorder most often resulting in homelessness. Schizophrenia is typically treated with medication, but people afflicted with schizophrenia often fail to take their medication due to distorted thinking about the reason it may have been prescribed (or a lack of belief it was needed).

This is why having a concrete support system is invaluable to those with schizophrenia. However, since many people of color face disparity in stable working hours, income, and treatment, this support is harder to find than with white patients.

Black and Brown families with a schizophrenic family member are often unable to receive mental health services to avoid an altercation resulting in the arrest of the schizophrenic person. If schizophrenia emerged in adolescence (which is common), the family burden for legal responsibility of the schizophrenic offspring's actions can quickly become overwhelming.

Meanwhile, race-based disparities in the diagnosis and treatment of people stricken with schizophrenia are evident.[120]

White people of higher socioeconomic status can utilize private mental health inpatient facilities (and all other psychiatric services) for their family members with schizophrenia far more easily than people of color. For this reason, white schizophrenics are anticipated to spend significantly less time in prison than Black and Brown schizophrenics.

Indeed, some can hold jobs and function well independently. Due to the large-scale closure of inpatient mental health facilities, lack of adequate health insurance, and reduced state funding for mental health services (including admission into residential halfway house settings), schizophrenics of color are most likely to become entangled in both the juvenile justice and adult prison systems.[121]

The "warehousing" of Black and Brown people with mental illness in the prison system not only worsens mental illness symptoms but negatively impacts the entire prison population.

As if this was not bad enough, a research article in *Psychiatric Services* in 2018 reported that Black and Brown people are five times more likely than whites to be diagnosed with schizophrenia and also have an elevated chance of being misdiagnosed with schizophrenia.[122]

The Disparate Impact of Substance Use Disorder on Communities of Color

One medical research article concluded the following. In comparison to the white population, African Americans have greater rates of illegal drug use and similar rates of alcohol abuse.

However, Latinx drug *and* alcohol rates are similar to that of the white population.[123]

While a link between drug addiction and socioeconomic status is described, what is missing is that, historically, organized crime syndicates led by white criminals flooded communities of color with illegal drugs so that white drug dealers would be less suspected.[124]

There is a strong relationship between mental illness, substance abuse disorder, and incarceration. Whether substance abuse disorder or mental illness came first can be disputed. However, those addicted to narcotics (*e.g.*, heroin and opioids) are typically unable to kick their habits without help.

More than 41% of African Americans have struggled with substance dependency, and 4% are heroin-addicted (per the US Substance Abuse and Mental Health Services Administration [SAMHSA]), and most of this subpopulation has struggled with a drug dependency.[125]

This is compared to 39.5% of Latinx people (with huge variations depending upon geographic location and origin).[126]

Alcohol abuse is common among Native Americans, but substance abuse disorder is less common in Asian communities.

While cocaine and prescription opioid abuse has historically been more prominent among whites than people of color (due to the elevated cost of cocaine and prescription opioids rivaled to other drugs), people of color are more subject to be arrested, receive a guilty verdict, be imprisoned, and receive a longer sentence than white people.

The federal guidance to states rendered in 2019 by the Trump Administration to require Medicaid recipients to work at least twenty hours each week or lose Medicaid coverage is especially harmful to adult heroin and opioid addicts participating in programs to halt their drug abuse. Fortunately, this federal Medicaid change has been stalled.[127]

While private insurance may cover participation in a program (whether inpatient or outpatient) to halt substance use disorder, public insurance does not cover anything except emergency detox in a hospital. This means that following a hospital stay of a day or two, heroin and opioid users receive no further support, so they are likely to relapse to drug use.

Meanwhile, a detoxed heroin user is susceptible to overdosing on the same amount of the drug that was previously a maintenance dose due to the build-up of physical tolerance. Therefore, heroin and opioid abusers are more vulnerable to overdose following detoxification.

Of course, a bad batch of an injectable street drug is just as likely to result in fatality. Either way, the lack of available substance abuse disorder treatment services to addicts, and particularly to heroin/opioid addicts of color, results in needless fatalities.

Although the foremost focus has been on the rise in overdose deaths among white users (and national opioid use rates are indeed raised for whites than they are for Black and Brown people), the rates of opioid deaths among Black and Brown individuals have been increasing. In many states, overdose deaths among African Americans actually exceed that of whites despite a lower use rate.

The avoidance of discussion around the opioid impact on the Black community is, whether intentional or not, promoting increased African American marginalization. Moreover, it highlights the historical nature of criminalizing addiction. By criminalizing addiction, people with substance abuse disorders are depicted as deserving punishment more than treatment.

To compound the problem, there are disparities in medication-assisted treatment (MAT) for African Americans, with white people 35% more likely than African Americans to receive MAT as hospitalized patients.

Two foremost barriers to substance abuse treatment are accessibility and insurance. The majority of patients who are not Black or Brown pay cash or use insurance. Only 25% of such encounters are covered by Medicaid or Medicare.

Thus, these two factors create unnecessary roadblocks to treatment. According to a 2017 report of the US Agency for Healthcare Research and Quality (AHRQ), "Overall access to efficient health care was worse for blacks than whites."

In addition, this report stated that "20% of Asian Americans, 30% of Native Americans, and a third of Pacific Islanders and Hispanics have access to effective healthcare."[128]

Impoverished Black and Brown people are the least likely to have access to either mental health services or substance abuse disorder treatment services. Not only does this impact the Black and Brown individuals, but it affects their children, who are subsequently at risk of developing a mental health and/or substance abuse disorder problem later in life.

African Americans who inject heroin also have a more increased risk of becoming infected with HIV/AIDS than either other African Americans or the US population at large. Not only are heroin and opioid abusers predisposed to dismal overall health resultant from their drug abuse lifestyle (including malnutrition and susceptibility to infection), but they are more likely to be homeless.

Since homelessness is more widespread among those of color than white people, Black and Brown injection drug users (including pregnant women) are also at increased risk for homelessness.

Disparity in Post-Traumatic Stress Disorder (PTSD) Between People of Color and White People

The prevailing incidence of PTSD in military veterans is well-known, and 22.6% of the total veteran population were people of color in 2014 (US Department of Veterans Affairs, 2017). This report also noted that 52% of minority veterans were African American, and 32% were Latinx.[129]

Meanwhile, PTSD can also result from exposure to neighborhood and domestic violence. Additionally, police-perpetrated violence toward African Americans and the Trump Administration's persistent targeting of Mexican Americans as the primary cause of crime across the US has also exacerbated PTSD in Black and Brown people.

This was also true before the beginning of the Covid-19 pandemic, which has promoted a spike in PTSD in people of color in the US.

PTSD is a condition that occurs in people who have suffered through traumatic events. It is normal for people to feel extremely anxious, frightened, or uncomfortable when facing situations that remind them of their traumatic experiences.

The Black community (and especially Black men) are dealing with some form of unresolved trauma related to inequitable treatment (whether in terms of employment, education, health, the criminal justice system, among others) that enforce the structures that cultivate and foster systematic racism.

Meanwhile, the lack of trust for law enforcement officers is yet another PTSD trigger, such as when Black and Brown people are pulled over while driving automobiles or just approached by culturally insensitive officers. Is it any wonder we become anxious and uncomfortable?

Indeed, this creates a perfect storm for Black and Brown people involving interactions with law enforcement members, especially those who are intolerant, racist, or culturally incompetent *and* lack de-escalation and crisis intervention training.

This applies to the discussion of mental health issues, as racism is a public health crisis that fully does evoke both physical and mental illness. I will discuss the impact of psychological stress on one's overall health in the next section.

Children who have witnessed domestic violence, undergone abuse (and especially sexual abuse), or have been exposed to violence around them are also more likely to develop PTSD. Moreover, a parent suffering from PTSD is more disposed to have offspring who develop PTSD.

The cycle continues through the generations, and it is all preventable since the causes of PTSD are societally inflicted. There is also far less treatment available for PTSD for people of color than for white people, so recovery is rendered more complex.

This discussion of PTSD was placed at the end of this section since there is a strong link between substance abuse disorder and PTSD.

As a mental health disorder, PTSD is the consequence of trauma, and that trauma can be inflicted on either an individual or an entire neighborhood. Systemic racism is the cause of so much of the PTSD in Black and Brown communities.

Nobody is born with PTSD. That is indeed the point!

I am concluding this section with the following quote that, for me, sums up how our society as a whole need to lessen the preventable high level of PTSD in Black and Brown communities.

"The fact is racism is producing a truly rigged system that is systematically disadvantaging some racial groups in the United States. To paraphrase Plato: There is nothing unfair as the equal treatment and unequal people. And that's why I am committed to working to dismantle racism." — David R. Williams (Professor of Public Health and Chair of the Department of Social and Behavioral Sciences at the Harvard University School of Public Health)

The Mental Health Link to Physical Health Outcomes

There is a well-recognized connection between psychological well-being and physical health outcomes. People who suffer from persistent depression and anxiety are more likely to experience poor physical health. One reason is that psychological stress depresses the immune system, thereby increasing the risk of both infection and inflammation (*e.g.*, intestinal inflammation).

Clinical depression is also explicitly connected to worse health outcomes because people who are depressed are less likely to acquire preventive healthcare and perform self-care to prevent chronic disorders from developing or worsening.

Meanwhile, anxiety promotes the body's release of adrenalin (a hormone that raises heart rate and blood pressure as part of the innate "fight or flight" response). When anxiety is prolonged, this can lead to high blood pressure, abnormal heart rhythm, and a hormonal-induced state of exhaustion.

Some disorders (such as Crohn's disease) are connected to psychological stress, and afflicted people often have more diarrhea when stressed. Disturbed sleep patterns and insomnia are often associated with bouts of depression.

In turn, poor quality sleep can lower immunity and foster a depressed mood. Meanwhile, the frequency of migraine headaches is also often raised in people experiencing psychological stress.

According to Duke Clinical Research Institute, a medical research study in 2015 focused on African American heart failure patients concluded a relationship between depression in study patients to worse cardiac outcomes.[130]

Indeed, tending to mental health is essential for physical health, while worsened mental health can lead to deteriorated overall health quality. The increased focus by physicians and nurses over the past twenty years on providing holistic healthcare results from longstanding medical research that unequivocally shows there *is* a "mind-body" connection.

Public health prevention includes caring for our mental health! However, the stigma attached to mental disorders promotes fear of seeking treatment. As a member of the African American community, I have personally known this fear.

American author, journalist and teacher, Bebe Moore Campbell, states that *"People of color, particularly African Americans, feel the stigma more keenly. In a race-conscious society, some don't want to be perceived as having yet another deficit."*

I definitely felt that. Let me pause to tell you my story.

On January 16, 2014, my father unexpectedly passed away. I was devastated and debilitated by fear, anxiety, and depression. Although I went to work every day (smiling and pretending to be okay), I experienced ever more difficulty living in my own skin. Being alone felt unbearable; I suffered in silence, and eventually, the silence became deafening.

Throughout that time, I pretended to be fine even though every moment of my life was consumed with the fear of death (which pushed me into severe anxiety attacks and bouts of depression that I think of as "grief attacks"). Meanwhile, I was terrified of being discovered and judged for my emotional turmoil.

I felt that I could not allow others to know that I was suffering to such a degree. One reason was that I did not want anyone to think I was incapable of performing my job since my career was on an upswing. In other words, I felt that I could not afford to have anyone doubting my abilities.

Whether consciously or not, I grasped that there was a horrible stigma attached to mental illness. As a God-fearing Black woman, I was taught not to claim things of this nature. Instead, I was told to take it to the Lord in prayer.

Therefore, I had to always be psychologically resilient because too many people depended on me to keep it together. Consequently, I suffered in silence and just dealt with it.

One year after my father's death, I lost my maternal grandmother. Then three weeks following this death, I lost my mother's brother. This was far too much for my heart to take (and, more significantly, my fragile mind to bear). Although I had suffered three considerable losses in a thirteen-month time frame, I did not want to seek help.

Yet, I could no longer suffer alone because the silence was too loud in my mind. I was then reminded that when my mother was in her early forties, she had suffered from depression climaxing in a mild nervous breakdown. I knew then I had to seek help.

Over the years since my father's death, I have become aware of many Black and Brown people (both young and old) who committed suicide because they had suffered alone in silence. This is a terrible tragedy, and I mourn their loss.

My main point in telling you all of this is to emphasize that we must remove the stigma from mental illness. We must encourage our family members and friends not to just pray but to actively seek help.

God has blessed many mental health professionals with the abilities and skill-sets to help us get through the most challenging times in life, and people of color have the same right and responsibility to seek help when overwhelmed in life.

I still struggle with fear, anxiety, and depression from time to time. However, I never want to be in a place in my mind again where the silence is too loud.

Therefore, I am openly telling you my story in hopes that this will enable others experiencing a mental health crisis to get help and not suffer alone! Let's help one another while helping ourselves! That's my heart's desire.

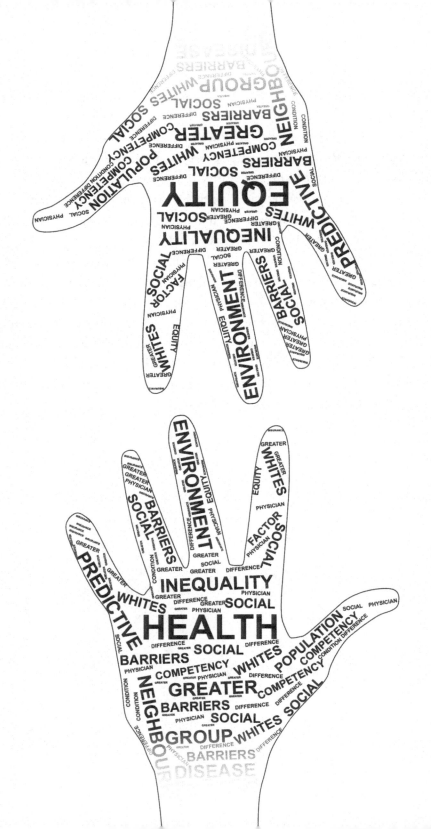

CHAPTER 10

Δ

JAIL AND PRISON POPULATIONS AND HEALTHCARE ACCESS

Access to healthcare is extremely limited in jails and prisons. It is crucial to recognize that prisoners in the US had a disproportionately high prevalence of infectious diseases, even before the Covid-19 pandemic commenced.[131]

Therefore, a substantial inequity exists between prisoners' access to healthcare and the non-imprisoned US population. African Americans are incarcerated in state prisons across the nation at more than five times the rate of whites.[132]

Most of the people arrested and subsequently sentenced to state prison are African American. Furthermore, Latinx people are incarcerated at a rate of 1.4% more than that of whites.[133]

Nearly 2.3 million people were incarcerated in the US as of 2017, and the US is foremost in the world in incarceration rates.[134]

Moreover, the rate of incarceration in the US has quadrupled in the past twenty-five years.[135] The privatization of prison healthcare began under President Reagan and multiplied over the next thirty years.[136]

At present, most healthcare services provided to prisoners are from for-profit companies rather than a public entity. This has not only decreased the quality of healthcare services (such as it was!) but increased the costs.

It has also enabled physicians and other clinicians who are not accountable to governmental entities but only to their companies at the helm of providing prisoner medical and psychiatric care.

For the incarcerated Black and Brown population, this leads to poorer health outcomes due to limited to no preventive screening, untreated symptoms, misdiagnosing, potentially more likely to recommend different routes of care that are more profitable for their company even if it sacrifices the health of the patient.

Meanwhile, incarcerated people are disproportionately from impoverished backgrounds. Black and Brown people living in poverty are unduly afflicted with chronic health conditions and are more likely to have weakened immune systems.

Therefore, Black and Brown prisoners are at a significant disadvantage in terms of health status *when arriving* for their imprisonment.

As mentioned previously, a grand proportion of incarcerated people in US jails and prisons live with a mental illness and/or have a substance abuse disorder. Prison deteriorates mental health and is even worse for someone already coping with a mental illness (*e.g.*, schizophrenia).

While incarceration has aided some drug-addicted people to stop abusing drugs while incarcerated, if they survive the terrible withdrawal symptoms typical of the "cold turkey" withdrawal approach, most incarcerated substance users return to their addiction upon release from prison.

The reason is that prisons do not offer substance disorder treatment, so a substance abuser who leaves prison to return to their former support system (typically other substance abusers) is likely to relapse.

According to the *International Journal of Prisoner Health*, prisoners in the US have a disproportionately high prevalence of infectious diseases, including viral hepatitis, HIV/AIDS, other sexually transmitted diseases, and tuberculosis.[137]

Indeed, HIV prevalence in US prisoners is around five times that of the general adult population (per a research article in 2017 in *AIDS Care*).[138]

The median incidence of tuberculosis among incarcerated people was twenty-nine cases per 100,000 local jail inmates, eight per 100,000 state prisoners, and twenty-five per 100,000 federal prisoners (per an article in the *American Journal of Public Health* in 2016).[139]

That is a lot of preventable diseases among prisoners!

In particular, HIV/AIDS (and other sexually transmitted diseases) are widespread among people who inject drugs such as heroin. Due to the large rate of sexual abuse among prisoners, the rate of HIV transmission (as well as other sexually transmitted diseases) is also more frequent than among the non-incarcerated population.

Meanwhile, around 4-6% of tuberculosis cases reported in the US are in incarcerated people diagnosed at the time of entry into incarceration.[140] Adherence to the daily antiretroviral drugs needed to prevent HIV/AIDS symptoms (and limit the potential for transmission) is difficult in the prison setting.

This promotes the potential for the emergency of drug-resistant HIV strains that can impact everyone on Earth who is HIV-positive.

Inequities in healthcare access for Black and Brown people are magnified in prison. A diabetes diagnosis requires controlling sugar intake to maintain health, but meals for prisoners tend to be low-quality, and exceptions are rarely made for prisoners with specific dietary needs.

Likewise, crowded housing conditions place the entire prison population at risk of infection, and most prisoners already have decreased immunity, putting them at higher risk of becoming ill.

The number of healthcare clinicians to inmates in jails and prisons is abysmally low.

For example, in Virginia in 2014, the ratio was forty physicians to 30,000 inmates.[141] Furthermore, physicians working in the penal system tend to be more recent graduates of medical schools (which is the main reason they sought employment in the prison system rather than elsewhere).

However, nurses are the primary healthcare providers in correctional facilities (per an article in *Implementation Science*).[142]

Mental Illness and Solitary Confinement

Solitary confinement is the primary "treatment" for an inmate with mental illness who is symptomatic. It is well-recognized that solitary confinement often results in psychological disturbances for anyone kept for more than twenty-four hours in such a cell.

Therefore, the use of solitary confinement to temporarily separate mentally ill prisoners from the rest of the prison population usually exacerbates their symptoms, resulting in a return with an extended stay in the solitary cell.

Schizophrenic inmates (exhibiting signs of paranoid schizophrenia) and receiving no treatment for their mental illness can also threaten the other prisoners' physical survival.

Since most prisoners are eventually released from prison, the pervasive lack of mental health treatment for psychiatrically disordered inmates raises the risk of them repeating the behavior that caused their arrest (and subsequent imprisonment) in the first place.

The Burden Placed on Prisoners of Color—Impact of Incarceration on Prisoners' Children

The massive disparity in incarceration rates resulting in such a dominant number of imprisoned Black and Brown people generates a burden for the families of these adults.

Notably, children with an incarcerated parent are three-fold more likely to exhibit behavioral problems and/or become clinically depressed, and they are two-fold more likely to have learning disabilities and Attention Deficit Hyperactivity Disorder (ADHD).[143]

When a parent becomes incarcerated, the entire family is affected. Black and Brown mothers are substantially more likely to be jailed than white mothers, and incarceration for a pregnant woman has a higher likelihood of terminating in newborn death.

Therefore, prisons are unsafe places for pregnant women while also creating irreparable damage to the relationship between the incarcerated mother and her children.

Incarceration and Likelihood of Worsened Future Health

Prisoners who develop cancer while in prison are far less likely to be treated at an early stage. Therefore, prisoners are more prone to developing inoperable cancer prior to their sentence completion.[144]

Due to the widespread prevalence of chronic HPV infection, women in prison are far more susceptible to developing uterine cancer than the general population.[145]

In the same vein, women with early-stage breast cancer are more *unlikely* to receive a rapid diagnosis (enabling potential treatment).

Covid-19 is shining a spotlight on the terrible conditions in US prisons contributing to decreased health status among incarcerated people. Many outbreaks in prisons across the nation have occurred and spread quickly throughout the entire inmate population.

The infection rate for prisoners in Washington, DC jails (as of May 2020) was fourteen times higher than for the rest of the city.[146]

Many US prisons started utilizing quarantine and solitary confinement to separate inmates testing positive for Covid-19 from the rest of the inmate population, but this has been met with widespread opposition from prisoners as it is akin to punishment for the misfortune of becoming infected.

Many US prisons started utilizing quarantine and solitary confinement to separate inmates testing positive for Covid-19 from the rest of the inmate population, but this has been met with widespread opposition from prisoners as it is akin to punishment for the misfortune of becoming infected.[147]

The consequence of the sorry state of medical care for prisoners is that many prisoners really have been given a death sentence regardless of the length of their original sentence.

Since adult children often want to aid their ill parents despite incarceration, lack of healthcare services to prisoners can place a substantial financial burden on adult children, elderly parents, and other family members. And these loved ones are often Black and Brown people who did nothing to deserve this burden.

Nothing so clearly demonstrates the inequity in healthcare access between people of color and the white population more than the mistreatment by the US prison healthcare system.

As prisoners are predominantly Black and Brown and locked in facilities removed from general public consciousness, maltreatment becomes easier.

CHAPTER 11

Δ

US MILITARY AND VETERANS' HEALTHCARE

It can take more time to acquire an appointment to see a healthcare provider in a Veterans Administration (VA) facility than in a non-*VA* facility.[148]

However, the problem is tremendously magnified for veterans seeking mental health and/or substance use disorder care. There is widespread acknowledgment that veterans (especially those who served in Vietnam, Afghanistan, and Iraq) have soaring rates of depression, anxiety, PTSD, and alcohol/drug dependence.[149]

Yet, it is hard for veterans to access either mental health or substance use disorder services.[150] Since so many veterans of US-initiated wars over the past fifty years are people of color, this is yet another racial disparity impacting overall health that needs to be recognized.

Suicide rates among veterans are 1.5 times that of non-veterans, so mental health services are certainly needed.[151] According to a publication in 2019 by the US Veterans Administration, homeless veterans are at the highest risk of suicide.[152]

This publication also noted that 58.7% of veterans who committed suicide in 2017 had a diagnosed mental illness or substance use disorder as of 2016 or 2017.

Unlike in the past, the multiple deployments to combat zones required of military personnel assigned to serve in Iraq and Afghanistan are recognized as contributing to the extraordinarily predominant intentional self-harm and suicidal ideation rates.

There are substantially more male veterans than female veterans, and suicide completion (versus suicide attempt) is recognized as more common in males who engage in a suicide attempt.

Furthermore, males attempting suicide are far more likely to use a firearm to complete suicide, which is one of the primary reasons males attempting suicide are more successful in their attempts. In contrast, females are more likely to self-poison by overdose, so they are more capable of receiving emergency medical care to reverse the effects.

Education, Civilian Job, and Social Support—
The Link to Veterans' Mental Health

In 2017, an article in the *International Journal of Mental Health Systems* noted that in recent years, the main reasons given for enlisting in the military are as follows: patriotism, educational benefits, a family tradition of military service, and financial inducements.[153]

For a sizeable number of youths of color, joining the military can appear to be a ticket to a better life.

This is especially the case for Black and Brown youths who do not have a viable path toward attending college. Such youths are most often from impoverished families, where they have no family role models for achieving more than a high school education.

Therefore, the capacity to acquire new skills that might later be applicable in civilian life can seem attractive, as well as the myriad of benefits for veterans offered by the federal government (including Veterans Administration [VA] loans for home-buying).

Military recruiters particularly target minority high school students to join the military, using some of the same marketing techniques employed by high-pressure car salespeople to convince the dealership visitor to buy a car!

Problematically, 35% of all veterans of color have a high school diploma or less as their highest level of educational attainment.[154]

Upon leaving the military, veterans who have developed a mental health disorder, such as PTSD or alcohol/drug dependence, may find it difficult to hold a job.

Meanwhile, veterans with low educational attainment may feel that their potential to improve their socioeconomic status is nil. Consequently, veterans of color from impoverished backgrounds with low educational attainment are at heightened risk for worsened mental health as veterans.

Veterans who lived a long distance from the nearest Veterans Administration Medical Center (VAMC) faced an additional hurdle in acquiring mental health and/or substance use disorder treatment services.

Since receiving mental health counseling or substance abuse disorder treatment can involve one or more weekly appointments, distance from the nearest VAMC creates an additional barrier on top of the long wait time to acquire services.

However, as of 2019, veterans can utilize non-VAMC services as long as they can show that the nearest VAMC is at least a thirty-minute drive from their residential address.[155]

Rather the entire system regarding how our health is covered prefers to benefit the white population.

Meanwhile, a *RAND* research brief in 2019 suggested that veterans received more appropriate mental health services from clinicians within the VA health system (due to familiarity with the issues faced by military personnel and veterans) than from mental health therapists and psychologists at non-VAMC sites.[156]

However, the truth is, these issues do not only affect veterans or impoverished people. Rather the entire system regarding how our health is covered prefers to benefit the white population. We will discuss this further in Part III.

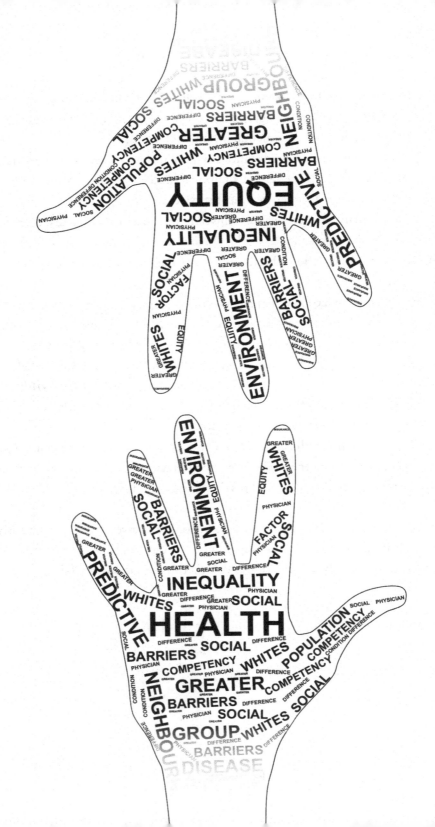

PART II

QUESTIONS TO PROMOTE YOUR THOUGHTS, KNOWLEDGE, AND SELF-AWARENESS

1. Have you ever felt that you were discriminated against based on race in a healthcare setting? If so, what happened, and how did this make you feel?

_____

_____

_____

_____

_____

2. If you are a person of color who has received care from a white physician (or other medical provider), do you feel that a white medical provider ever made stereotyped assumptions about your background and interests? If so, how did this make you feel?

_____

_____

_____

_____

_____

3. If you are not a person of color, have you ever felt that you were treated differently in a healthcare setting because you were white (rather than a person of color)? If you have had an experience (or more than one) of preferential treatment based on race, how did it make you feel?

_____

_____

_____

_____

_____

4. Have you ever felt that you needed support for your mental health? If so, did you reach out for such support, and did you receive it?

_____

_____

_____

_____

_____

5. If you have ever received psychological counseling, do you feel that the counseling met your needs? Why, or why not?

_____

_____

_____

_____

_____

6. Have you ever felt that you needed support for a dependence on alcohol, drugs, or other substance? If so, did you seek such support, and did you receive it?

_____

_____

_____

_____

_____

7. Have you or anyone you know received inappropriate psychological or substance abuse disorder services, and what occurred? If you (or someone you know) is a person of color, do you feel that the inappropriate services would have been *less* inappropriate if you (or they) were not a person of color?

_____

_____

_____

_____

_____

8. If you are a healthcare professional or mental health professional who is a person of color, have you ever felt that you were treated in a prejudicial manner by a supervisor, colleague, or patient/client because you were a person of color? How did this make you feel?

_____

_____

_____

9. Have you (or someone you know) ever spent any time in jail or prison? Did this impact your feelings about yourself (or the other person who was imprisoned)? How did the imprisonment affect your life and/or the life of someone else you know who was imprisoned?

_____

_____

_____

_____

_____

10. Are you (or anyone you know) actively serving in the US military or a US military veteran? If so, and you are a person of color, do you feel that you were treated differently as either an active military member or a veteran? How do you feel about the healthcare services and/or mental health services you have received as an active military member or veteran?

_____

_____

_____

_____

_____

PART III

Health Insurance Coverage Inequities

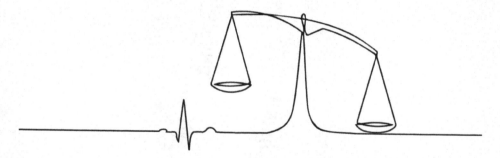

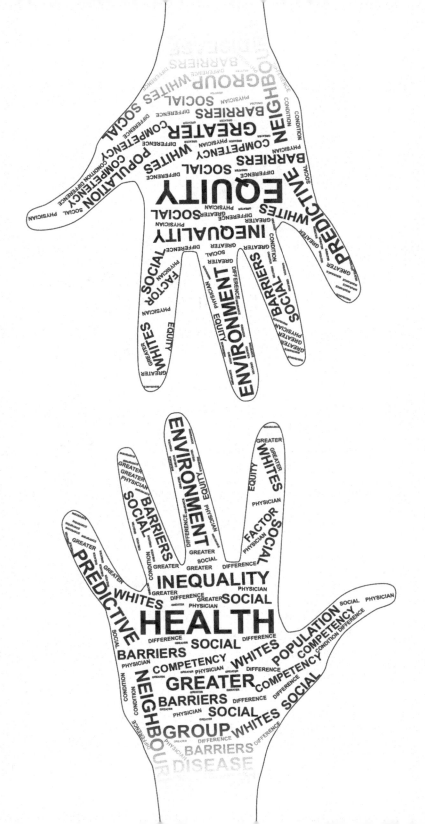

CHAPTER 12

Δ

WHY HEALTH INSURANCE IS KEY TO QUALITY HEALTHCARE AT PRESENT

Hospitals, outpatient healthcare providers, and rehab centers all depend upon health insurance payments for the main proportion of their revenue stream. How many people do you know that self-pay for all of their hospitalization and rehab costs?

Probably nobody. Not even the executive management staff of top-earning US technology companies normally pay for all of their healthcare "out-of-pocket."

Some millionaires from other countries specifically visit the US for their medical care and are self-paying (referred to as *medical tourists*), *providing* extra dollars for hospitals and specialty practices. However, consider that the average cost for a liver transplant is $812,500, not including hospital room and physician charges.[157]

This may give you a picture of the level of accessible cash often required of medical tourists for treatment in the US.

The following are some statistics to consider if you are an employed US resident and have the shortsighted urge to drop your health insurance to save money for a future vacation.

Hospital costs in the US in 2017 averaged $3,949 per day (with a hospital stay expense average of $15,734).[158] The average cost of an uncomplicated appendectomy is $33,000.[159]

The current reality is that due to the astronomical cost of healthcare in the US, 60% of all personal bankruptcies in the US are the result of medical bills *overwhelming* a person's financial resources.[160] One medical crisis is really all it takes!

Admission to a hospital for a non-emergency surgery is not likely if you do not have health insurance coverage or do not have *adequate* health insurance coverage. The staff at outpatient physician practices typically ask for the type of insurance coverage before scheduling an appointment.

60% of all personal bankruptcies in the US are the result of medical bills overwhelming a person's financial resources. One medical crisis is really all it takes!

Many will no longer accept new Medicare and/or Medicaid patients as the reimbursement rates are generally lower than from private insurance companies, close to five cents on every dollar.

However, this longstanding practice is shifting somewhat due to the national move to value-based payment models, as these are focused on quality outcomes.

For example, Comprehensive Care Plus (CPC+) is an advanced Patient Care Medical Home (PCMH) model focused on strengthening primary care services through payment reform transformation of how care is delivered. Comprehensive Primary Care (CPC) is Medicaid's patient PCMH program.

Notably, a team-based care delivery model is led by a Primary Care Physician (PCP) to provide comprehensive, holistic care.

Whether recovery after hospitalization is in a rehab center or with home-based nursing or clinical therapy assistance, a person discharged from a hospital without the requisite health insurance coverage may not be able to get the care needed to fully recuperate following discharge (*i.e.,* leaving the hospital after such health-affecting events as joint replacement surgery, pneumonia, or a stroke).

According to the Kaiser Family Foundation (*KFF*), most uninsured people do not receive health services for free or at a reduced charge. Indeed, only 27% of uninsured adults in 2015 reported receiving services for free or at a decreased cost.

Furthermore, uninsured people often must pay out-of-pocket in advance before receiving any healthcare services.[161]

Adding to the burden placed on uninsured patients, the invoice received is often for the total cost of the services (as opposed to a potentially negotiated discounted bill submitted to insurers).[162]

Is it any wonder that so many people in the US are terrified of not having adequate health insurance in case of need?

Impact of *the Affordable Care Act* (ACA)

The Center on Budget and Policy Priorities (CBPP) reported that the *Affordable Care Act* (ACA) enabled twenty million more people to gain health insurance than before its passage.

While 50% of the increased people covered by insurance was due to access to private health insurance, the rest was due to the following three occurrences: the ability of young people to remain on their parents' health plans until age twenty-six; prevention of insurers' legal capacity to refuse coverage due to a pre-existing health condition; and the ACA-enacted Medicaid expansion.[163]

Let's pause for a moment. It is important to understand that the ACA Medicaid Expansion allowed states to cover their low-income residents up to 138% of the Federal Poverty Level (FPL).[164]

Many low-income people work in retail and manual labor jobs without employer-based insurance coverage and earn more than the FPL. However, they do not earn enough to enable the self-purchase of health insurance.

This is one of the reasons why Medicaid expansion was vital for these working adults to be able to see doctors when needed.

Additionally, noted by the CBPP report was that the rate of uninsured Americans fell precipitously across all of the following four tracked demographics after the passage of the ACA: income, age, race/ethnicity, and education.

For African Americans, the level of health insurance numbers of insured adults in the US population remained below that of Latinx, Asian, and white citizens but was still dramatically increased.[165]

In summary and according to a Brookings Institute article in 2020, "Since the ACA's core coverage provision came into effect in 2014, uninsured rates fell across all racial and ethnic groups, with the biggest gains among Black and Hispanic people."[166]

In 2017, private health insurance coverage for the US population as a whole continued to be more prevalent than government-provided health insurance (at 67% and 38%, respectively), and employer-based health insurance predominated at 56%, followed by Medicaid at 19%.[167]

The attempts to repeal and replace the ACA under the Trump presidency have resulted in a decreased number of people in the US covered by health insurance. This is a real setback toward the goal of insurance coverage for all US residents that places yet another burden on President Biden's administration.

In particular, the states that did not participate in the Medicaid expansion, all of which had Republican governors, left many residents uninsured.[168]

Furthermore, between 2017 and 2018, two million people were uninsured (which was raised from 2016-2017).[169] This increase in total uninsured was consequent to restrictions imposed on the ACA per the national healthcare policy documents of President Trump and his cabinet appointee (head of the DHHS).[170]

The Problem of High-Deductible Health Plans for Accessing Healthcare

Adults without employer-based health insurance coverage—under the ACA—can purchase insurance under the federal exchanges categorized as "gold," "silver," and "bronze." While "silver" and "bronze" plans are less expensive than "gold" plans, the disadvantage is that they have more costly annual deductibles.

This means that the dollar amount specified as the deductible (*e.g.*, $1000) needs to be paid out-of-pocket by the insured person before the insurance plan will cover the insured person's healthcare expenses.

Since people of color are disproportionately prone to have lower income (whether employed or self-employed), more "silver" and "bronze" plans have been chosen by African Americans and Latinx people for purchase on the ACA exchanges since the premium (monthly cost to the enrollee for the selected insurance plan) is lower than for a "gold" plan.

However, as already mentioned, Black and Brown people are also more likely not to have employer-sponsored health insurance coverage.

Even for those people fortunate to have employer-paid health insurance, many are only offered enrollment in high-deductible plans, especially people working for small businesses (although it is important to know that small businesses with fifty or fewer employees are exempt from the ACA requirement to offer health coverage for their employees).[171]

Problematically, small businesses most often cannot afford to provide plans with lower deductibles as these tend to be more costly for employers.

Consequently, small business employees across the US, who are disproportionately Black and Brown people, are typically provided with high-deductible health insurance plans, so they avoid scheduling doctor's appointments unless absolutely needed.

In a nutshell, this is an introduction to health insurance issues that foster inequities in healthcare system utilization in general. These are crucial to grasp the "down-the-road" effect on healthcare access for people of color. But there is more to consider to comprehend the full picture of the impact.

Chronic Health Disorders — Relationship of Outcomes to Health Insurance Coverage

For people with chronic health disorders and high-deductible health plans, choosing to skip regular healthcare appointments may make short-term financial sense so that a mortgage or rent payment can be paid by the due date. However, skipping appointments can also have a detrimental effect on overall health status.

For example, kidney damage is a frequent consequence of many chronic disorders (*e.g.,* diabetes, various autoimmune diseases, and heart damage). Without a health check-up inclusive of routine lab tests, a person with kidney damage may not know the damage is progressing and, therefore, may not be started on a treatment regimen to reverse that damage.

The result may be an avoidable progression to total kidney failure and the permanent need for dialysis (to perform the blood-cleaning task of the failed kidneys).

For someone with early-stage cancer or an early-stage infection, not receiving medical care in a timely fashion can also result in dire consequences. Meanwhile, people who have to pay high deductibles (and/or high co-pays) can be so squeezed financially that they avoid treatment or medications that could significantly improve their quality of life.

For anyone with severe osteoarthritis needing a knee replacement, foregoing that surgery can mean an inability to walk. In turn, a reduced capacity to exercise can result in more health problems.

Choosing a health plan that only allows care by in-network providers is often less expensive than one allowing a more expansive choice of hospitals and physicians but being limited to in-network providers may not enable the best quality of healthcare for everyone.

This is especially the case in certain rural geographic areas where an in-network hospital or provider in a given health plan may be fifty or more miles away from the insured person's home.

Even for someone covered by traditional Medicare, which covers 80% of hospitalization and outpatient provider costs, the purchase of supplemental insurance (termed *Medigap* insurance) can make all the difference between seeking medical care and avoiding it since a *Medigap* plan may cover the cost of the 20% not covered by original Medicare.

Hospitalization statistics on the Covid-19 pandemic reveal the disparity between the health impact on Black and Brown people and everyone else. Since treatment (as opposed to testing) for Covid-19 was not covered for most people by the federal CARES Act, it is still unclear who will be responsible for the bill for that care.

However, the portion of the bill not covered by insurance is commonly passed to the person hospitalized. In this way, the healthcare inequity that Black and Brown people face in the US is exacerbated during this pandemic.

Even if an insured person just seeks physician care in the Emergency Department (ED) due to not having a Primary Care Provider (PCP)and is *not* admitted to the hospital, that ill person is likely to receive a bill since numerous Preferred Provider Organization (PPO) plans do not cover any visit to an ER deemed by the health plan not to be medically necessary.

Health Insurance and Mental Health/Substance Use Disorder Services

In 1995, the *Mental Health Parity and Addiction Equity Act* (MHPAEA) was enacted. According to the Centers for Medicare and Medicaid Services (CMS) website, this federal law "prevents group health plans and health insurance issuers that provide mental health or substance use disorder (MH/SUD) benefits from imposing less favorable benefit limitations on those benefits than on medical/surgical benefits."[172]

However, the reality is that many insurance companies are not in compliance with this law.[173]

According to a 2019 Milliman, documenting this widespread noncompliance, many people enrolled in PPOs that required higher co-insurance percentages from enrollees using out-of-network service did not provide parity for access to mental health service providers compared to service providers for physical health disorders.[174]

In other words, these PPOs make it less difficult to acquire services for solely physical ailments rather than psychiatric disorders.

Additionally, many insurance plans get away with something similar to noncompliance by determining a behavioral health service for an enrollee to be "not medically necessary."

For example, since a given enrollee does not know how many other enrollees have been denied inpatient behavioral health services as opposed to outpatient services, that enrollee may feel this is just an individual rather than a pervasive occurrence. That enrollee may also accept receiving outpatient services and not fight the decision when inpatient services are actually needed.

All too often, impatient services for someone with a psychiatric disorder are limited by a health insurance company to only a week or so, when an extended stay could provide the support needed by the affected person to prevent a near-term recurrence of psychiatric symptoms.

Lower-cost health insurance plans usually offer worse coverage for mental health and substance use disorder treatment, although this is not always the case, as each plan determines its own coverage parameters.

Meanwhile, for a person of color who needs mental health or substance use disorder counseling, the in-network providers may or may not possess any "cultural competence."

Only 5% of practicing psychologists in the US are African American,[175] and the American Psychological Association (APA) reports only around 5% are Latino/Hispanic.[176]

Nobody wants to see a therapist who is un-empathetic. However, white mental health/substance use disorder counselors may bring their own prejudiced attitudes to the clinician-client relationship. Is it any wonder that Brown and Black people who need mental health and/or substance use disorder counseling choose not to proceed?

Overall, health insurance inequities in the US foster healthcare access disparities that have particularly negative consequences for Black and Brown people. This also promotes differences between hospitals and healthcare providers primarily serving impoverished communities and those serving wealthier, typically "white-majority" ones.

In this current dysfunctional health insurance landscape, healthcare facilities serving primarily people of color are typically cash-strapped and, therefore, under-staffed.

The US healthcare system is not only *not* cost-effective, but it also fosters inequalities that contribute to worsened health outcomes for people who do not have top-notch health insurance coverage. And those people are all too often people of color.

CHAPTER 13

Δ

BIAS IN TREATMENT OF THE UNINSURED AND MEDICAID-INSURED IN THE US

Most people in the US covered by Medicaid, to the surprise of many white people, are white rather than people of color. Consider the following statistics. Of the sixty-eight million people aged nineteen to sixty-four covered by Medicaid in 2018, 46% were white.[177]

Meanwhile, 34% of Medicaid enrollees in 2018 were African American.[178] Notably, 37% of all adult Medicaid beneficiaries are working, and 34% are the parent of a dependent child.[179]

Furthermore, for the twenty-three million adults under sixty-five in the US with disabilities (such as caused by blindness or multiple sclerosis [MS]), Medicaid is the primary payer for essential long-term services and supports.[180]

As previously mentioned, it can be arduous for Medicaid-insured people to access outpatient healthcare services[181] since many payments to physicians by Medicaid can be less than by private insurers.

They are not "revenue-boosting" for healthcare clinicians, resulting in reluctance by physicians to accept Medicaid-insured patients.

Indeed, an article in 2018 in *BMC Health Services Research* stated, "Declining job satisfaction and concurrent reductions in Medicaid participation among primary care providers have been documented."[182]

According to the Medicaid and CHIP Payment and Access Commission (MACPAC), deferred medical care due to a healthcare access obstacle related to cost, provider-related reasons, and/or a lack of transportation was 14% for Medicaid-insured adults as opposed to only 8% for privately insured adults.[183]

Physician Attitudes Toward Their Medicaid Patients

Study findings the *Journal of Family Medicine* showed that 86% of the specialist physicians surveyed (most of whom were white) had an unfavorable perception of Medicaid-enrolled patients, with overall perceptions that Medicaid patients were "socially-complicated," "medically-complicated," and had "poor adherence to lifestyle recommendations."[184]

This article also noted that respondents generally agreed with the perspective that Medicaid patients were disreputable, unappreciative, and unaccountable and that these survey results mirrored study results for Primary Care Physicians [PCPs].

These co-authors concluded that some of the study outcomes linked to Medicaid patients, such as a greater likelihood of skipping appointments without canceling than privately insured patients, can be attributed to the socioeconomic determinants of health.

They also concluded that biased attitudes toward Medicaid patients by physicians could impact their medical treatment of them. Really, you think?

Existent Biases Toward Poor People Transferred to Medicaid Recipients

Pervasive biases toward poor people had been promoted in the US, including the belief that poor people are lazy and irresponsible. This is an outgrowth of the viewpoint promoted in K-12 schools that our nation is a classless society and that the American Dream is achievable by anyone with enough determination to pursue it.

In contrast, societal inequities exist that make it extremely difficult for specific subpopulations (such as low-income Black and Brown people) to successfully climb the socioeconomic ladder, as described in Part II of this book.

MACPAC reported that around 40% of all individuals enrolled in Medicaid in 2017 had family incomes below 100% of the Federal Poverty Level (FPL). So, extremely poor.[185]

To put this level of poverty in context, it can be difficult for someone living below 100% of the FPL to afford food and prescribed medication; therefore, many choose to stretch their medication rather than pay for more drugs in order to afford food.

A person living below 100% of the FPL is also unlikely to replace a car when it dies or acquire a credit card. These all contribute to being unable to avoid the development (or worsening) of a chronic health disorder.

While someone covered by private insurance who receives a denial of coverage for a service (*i.e.,* an MRI) may have the income to hire a lawyer to fight that denial, Medicaid enrollees seldom have the resources to fight a Medicaid coverage denial. And Medicaid tends to *not* cover anything it can legally avoid covering.

The Politics of Medicaid — Its Impact on Enrollees

Medicaid is a federal-state partnership, so states have a great deal of control over Medicaid-paid medical services in a given state.

Moreover, at least 66% of Medicaid-enrollees get care through privately managed care plans (and these typically limit their enrollees to receiving care solely through in-network providers).[186]

Another finding in the above-noted article in the *Journal of Family Medicine* showed 52% of the specialist physicians surveyed limited their acceptance of Medicaid-insured patients or no longer accepted Medicaid-insured patients.[187]

Federally Qualified Health Centers (FQHC) were created to deliver care to vulnerable individuals and families, and most receive *Health Center Program* federal grant funding to improve the care of underserved and vulnerable populations.[188]

They are more often found in mutually underserved areas (MUA). Due to persistent underfunding, the staff is typically underpaid and overworked. Therefore, many of the physicians are recent medical school graduates. However, they have a passion for the mission of caring for the sickest of the sick and the most vulnerable populations of people.

According to the National Association of Community Health Centers, public health centers provide primary care for more than one in every six Medicaid patients nationwide.[189]

In addition, some also provide dental, vision, mental health and substance use care, and pharmaceutical services. In 2019, the Trump Administration's budget called for a cut of more than $236 million for chronic disease promotion and health promotion,[190] which are vital areas of focus of FQHCs.

The federal government under President Trump approved state requirements for Medicaid recipients to work to qualify for Medicaid.

In 2018, that approval was granted to Arkansas, Indiana, Kentucky, and New Hampshire, with eight more states having pending waivers (per the Pew Charitable Trusts).[191]

However, the US Appeals Court for the District of Columbia Circuit in 2020 upheld the 2019 lower court ruling blocking states' Medicaid work requirements.[192]

Still, much damage was already done. In Arkansas, it caused thousands of Medicaid recipients to become dis-enrolled,[193] and whether all of these people were later re-enrolled remains unknown. As anyone who has ever completed the forms required to enroll (or renew enrollment) in Medicaid recognizes, the paperwork is time-consuming.

The principally Republican-led states that sought to enforce work requirements to remain on Medicaid showed an utter lack of recognition of the health factors that can prevent a Medicaid recipient from holding a job.

It involves the submission of various pieces of documentation (*e.g.,* copy of most recent IRS 1040 tax form, last three months of paystubs or other proof of income as well as utility bills, etc.).

Talk about insular perceptions. The principally Republican-led states that sought to enforce work requirements to remain on Medicaid showed an utter lack of recognition of the health factors that can prevent a Medicaid recipient from holding a job.

However, it is imperative to note that most Medicaid recipients are actually employed. For example, a diabetic may need frequent breaks to eat. A person with a degenerated lumbar spine disc may be unable to sit or stand for long periods, and a person who has experienced a car accident with brain injury may not be able to concentrate.

Relatedly, recovering substance abusers may need to participate in daily sessions with counselors to not relapse.

The problem for many people with chronic health conditions is that they may not be considered disabled enough to qualify for permanent benefits.

Yet, they still may be unable to hold (or acquire) regular employment due to the health disorder *or* (for someone chronically disabled who actually acquires a job) functioning in the workplace role may worsen their symptoms.

The past year of the current Covid-19 pandemic has demonstrated that treating Medicaid enrollees differently than other people in terms of healthcare access can foster community-wide spread of the virus. Since so many essential workers are Medicaid beneficiaries, it is even more important that inequity in access to services between Medicaid patients and privately insured patients be addressed.

Lack of Care for the Uninsured

In 2017, there were twenty-nine million uninsured people in the US,[194] and people of color were at the highest risk of being uninsured.[195]

Meanwhile, most uninsured people are in low-income families with at least one employed person in the family.[196] 7% of the total US population in 2018 were non-citizens, and four in every ten undocumented US resident was uninsured.[197]

Young adults across the demographic spectrum in the US are usually uninsured, as this age group tends to feel more invulnerable to becoming sick, so some forego health insurance to save money for preferred activities.

Whatever the reason, not having insurance leads to increased use of emergency rooms. Following the enactment of the ACA (with Medicaid expansion),

ER visits in 2016 by uninsured patients dropped nationally from 16% in 2006 to 8%.[198]

Hospitals and outpatient health centers alike are burdened when large numbers of uninsured patients need their care. This is because the hospitals and outpatient healthcare centers have to absorb the costs.

For hospitals and outpatient health centers serving huge numbers of uninsured people, the costs can become overwhelming (and this occurred before the ACA).

In 2021, the US Supreme Court will decide *Texas v. United States* to determine the constitutionality of the ACA, which will have tremendous implications for all US residents.[199]

For the sake of patients and healthcare providers alike, the US health system needs to be improved so that no one in the nation is uninsured or underinsured. Significant inequities exist in health insurance access, and this translates into access to healthcare services.

Yet again, such injustices have a disproportionately adverse effect on African American, Latinx, and Native American people.

PART III

QUESTIONS TO PROMOTE YOUR THOUGHT, KNOWLEDGE, AND SELF-AWARENESS

1. Do you have health insurance? If so, are you happy with your insurance plan? If not, why not?

_____

_____

_____

_____

_____

2. If you do not have health insurance, why not? How does this make you feel about making appointments for healthcare if you need them?

_____

_____

_____

_____

_____

3. If you have health insurance through an employer, did you have a choice of health insurance plan, or was only one insurance plan available from your employer? Do you feel that your current health insurance meets your needs? Why or why not?

_____

_____

_____

_____

_____

4. Do you ever worry about being able to pay a healthcare bill if you need to visit a doctor or become admitted to a hospital? If so, why? If not, why not?

_____

_____

_____

_____

_____

5. Have you (or anyone you know) ever been covered by Medicaid? If so, have you (or anyone you know) been treated *worse* for having Medicaid than private insurance? If so, what happened that made you believe this to be the case?

_____

_____

_____

_____

6. Have you (or anyone you know) not made an appointment for healthcare or not filled a drug prescription because of worry about the financial cost to you? If so, how did this make you feel?

_____

_____

_____

_____

_____

7. Have you (or anyone you know) filled a prescription for medication but skipped taking some pills due to worry about the financial cost to you? If so, how did this make you feel?

_____

_____

_____

_____

_____

8. Have you (or anyone you know) ever needed to *choose* between buying food or paying for prescription medication due to financial cost to you? If so, how did this make you feel?

_____

_____

_____

_____

_____

9. Have you ever not been able to see a healthcare provider you wanted to see because that provider did not accept your health insurance? How did this make you feel?

_____

_____

_____

_____

_____

10. If you have ever had to switch from a health insurance plan (such as due to moving to a different geographic area or starting a new job) that you liked to one that you liked *less*, what made you feel *less* happy with that new health insurance plan?

_____

_____

_____

_____

_____

11. Have you ever decided to get a health insurance plan because it appeared to cost less on a monthly or yearly basis? What made you decide to choose the less expensive health plan? After you enrolled in this health plan, did you feel that you made the right decision for yourself? Why, or why not?

_____

_____

_____

12. What would you do differently (if anything) in your life if you did not have to worry about *ever* having to pay a healthcare or hospital bill?

_____

_____

_____

_____

_____

13. Have you (or anyone you know) ever been unable to pay a doctor or hospital bill at the time it was due for payment? How did this make you feel?

_____

_____

_____

_____

14. If you are a person of color, have you ever felt that you were treated differently by a health insurance company (or a representative of that company) because of your race? If so, how did this make you feel?

_____

_____

_____

15. If you have health insurance, have you ever been denied coverage for something you felt that you needed because the insurance company said it was "not medically necessary"? If so, how did this make you feel, and what did you do about it?

_____

_____

_____

_____

_____

_____

PART IV
ADVOCATING FOR EQUITY

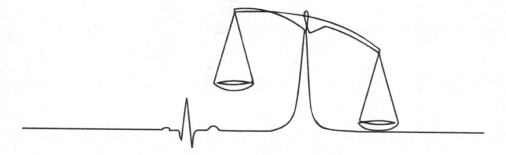

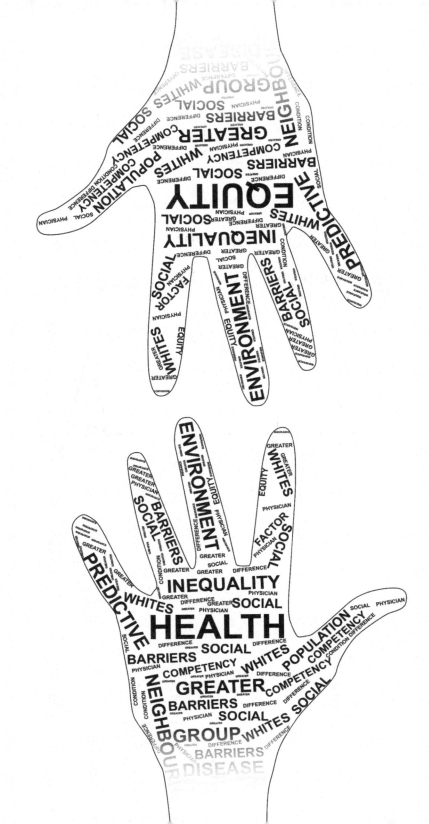

CHAPTER 14

Δ

WHAT THE COVID-19 PANDEMIC HAS REVEALED ABOUT DISPARITIES

In 2020, we faced two major public health crises in the US at the same time. One was racism (as discussed throughout this book); the other was the Covid-19 pandemic.

Both of these crises disproportionately have impacted Black and Brown people. As extensively described in Parts I through III of this book, the disparities faced by Black and Brown people have been perpetuated by systematic health and social inequities.

SDoH preventing opportunities for wellness and creating barriers to those opportunities must be eradicated. Meanwhile, the same issues related to the SDoH have contributed to the heightened risk for Black and Brown people to contract (and die from) a Covid-19 infection.

Globally, the coronavirus pandemic that began in January 2020 in Wuhan, China, has promoted a surge in awareness of the interdependence of everyone on Earth. A virus normally found in an animal jumped from an animal host to a human.

Before considering the impact of the pandemic in solely the US, let's consider first how an infection made this leap with a brief overview of Covid-19 from a historical perspective.

Understanding Covid-19 — A Brief History

Basically, humans and wildlife have never before lived in such proximity with each other. While *zoonotic* infections (which leap from animals to humans) are not a new phenomenon, this leap has been increasing over the past sixty years.

One of the primary reasons for the expedited emergence of zoonotic infections is the growing proximity of humans to wildlife as humans continue to encroach ever more on land formerly only occupied by wildlife, whether through worldwide population growth or ever-increasing worldwide urbanization.

In the case of SARS-CoV-2 (real name of Covid-19), an animal sold live and killed for sale at the outdoor Huanan Seafood Market in Wuhan started the chain of events and has affected all-too-many lives during this pandemic.

Due to widespread global airplane travel for business and leisure activities (along with international trade involving the widespread use of container ships along with airplanes), rapid transmission of the outbreak from Wuhan to some other parts of China and the rest of the globe was able to occur in record time.

Later in January 2020, Italy became the next epicenter of this outbreak (which fostered its spread to the rest of Europe and throughout the US). Meanwhile, Covid-19 mutated and became even more contagious.

On January 15, 2020, someone who had recently traveled overseas and then returned to Seattle, WA feeling ill, became the first person in the US who tested positive for Covid-19. A small outbreak occurred in the greater Seattle area.[200]

Around the same time, someone in California tested positive for Covid-19, and the first case in New York City was confirmed on March 1, 2020.[201]

It is important to note that the Covid-19 strain found in everyone except for a few early infected people in Washington and California is the mutated strain that emerged in Italy.

This is important because President Trump has repeatedly referred to Covid-19 as the "Chinese virus" or "Wuhan virus," which has fanned racist attitudes and activities toward Asian people across the US.

This is important because President Trump has repeatedly referred to Covid-19 as the "Chinese virus" or "Wuhan virus," which has fanned racist attitudes and activities toward Asian people across the US.[202] Presently, the most prevalent global strain is the UK (mutated) strain.

As of August 19, 2020, cases of Covid-19 in the US totaled five point fifty-five million, and 173,000 US residents had died from this infection. (As of February 24, 2021, 503,000 US residents have now died from this infection.) Even with the commencement of a nationwide vaccination effort, infections and deaths from Covid-19 are continuing to occur.

By the time you read this book, another 100,000 people across the US may have died of this rampantly contagious disease.

Other Zoonotic Infection Outbreaks Since Calendar Year 2000

Some nations fought recent zoonotic outbreaks before the Covid-19 pandemic, as described below:

In 2003, a viral outbreak of a new disease primarily affecting the upper respiratory tract occurred in China. It is widely believed by medical researchers to have originated in bats before transferring into civet cats and then into humans.

This coronavirus was termed SARS (*Severe Acute Respiratory Syndrome*). Before the SARS outbreak ended later in 2003, it had spread to twenty-six countries and had infected a reported 8,098 people, with 774 resulting deaths.[203]

In 2009, a coronavirus outbreak of "Swine Flu" occurred. It was caused by an H1N1 influenza strain that had never previously existed in humans (so no flu vaccine to protect against this strain was available for nineteen months).

The outbreak affected at least 214 countries, and 575,400 deaths were reported to the World Health Organization (WHO).[204]

In 2012 in Saudi Arabia, a coronavirus outbreak, MERS (*Middle East Respiratory Syndrome*), began. Outbreaks have since occurred in twenty-seven countries (with most cases occurring in the Middle East).

The MERS case fatality rate was 34%, measured up against a fatality rate for SARS of around 10%.[205]

Notably, Covid-19 is generally considered more easily transmissible (via airborne droplets) from one person to another but less fatal than either SARS or MERS.[206]

Besides the above-described recent coronavirus outbreaks, the zoonotic infection termed Ebola, which is spread primarily through direct contact with blood and body fluids, needs to be included in this presentation. Between 2014 and 2016, 28,000 people were infected in Africa (mostly in West Africa), and there were some cases diagnosed in Europe and the US.

The fatality rate after Ebola infection is 88%, making it the deadliest of the recent zoonotic infectious diseases.[207]

The last known outbreak of Ebola (before the current one in the Republic of Guinea and the Democratic Republic of Congo) was in 2020 in the Democratic Republic of Congo, and that outbreak was declared over by the WHO on June 25, 2020.[208]

Covid-19 in the US — Comparing Infection Rates by Race in the US

As of August 2020, the Centers for Disease Control noted reported cases of Covid-19 were nearly three-fold higher for African American, Latinx, and Native American people than for white people in the US, and hospitalization due to Covid-19 was nearly five-fold higher for African American and Latinx people (and 5.3 times higher for Native Americans) than for white people.[209]

The CDC also reported that the death rate from Covid-19 was African Americans (2.1 times higher than for whites), Latinx (1.1 times higher than for whites), Native Americans (1.4 times higher than for whites).

No significant difference was displayed in the rates between Asian people and white people in the US.[210]

According to the Commonwealth Fund in April 2020, "By April 21, large-concentration black communities saw 422,184 confirmed Covid-19 cases and 27,354 deaths, contrasted against 378,667 cases and 16,203 deaths in low-concentration black counties."[211]

Statistics reported by race all reveal that Covid-19 disproportionately impacts Black and Brown people. Moreover, Black and Brown people are more likely to die from contracting this virus.

Study findings from the APM Research Lab show the following: the death toll from Covid-19 for African Americans was 35,932 (as of August 18, 2020), representing the most dominant Covid-19 mortality rate of any ethnic group in the US. The APM Research Lab also presented a reported Latinx death toll of 32,538.[212]

However, this number may have been an undercount since many undocumented Latinx people (including permanent residents with an undocumented family member) may be fearful of any interaction with a US healthcare and/or governmental entity due to the intentionally cruel deportation climate under President Trump.

A report of the Marguerite Casey Foundation sums up the Covid-19 disparity by stating, "The pandemic is exposing racial disparities like few other events in recent U.S. history with initial data showing that Covid-19 is infecting and killing Black people at a far larger rate than any other group."[213]

Finally, the Mayo Clinic suggests the overall disparity in Covid-19 cases between whites and Black/Brown people may be due to a combination of the higher prevalence of chronic health disorders, usual work (occupation), and access to healthcare.[214]

As previously mentioned, Black and Brown people are disproportionately frontline workers, so more exposed to infection by Covid-19. The US political climate exacerbated by President Trump is adding to the difficulties facing Black and Brown working people.

Under Mitch McConnell's former Senate leadership, the extension of federal-subsidized unemployment benefits provided under the *CARES Act* was interrupted (since the Republican-controlled Senate wanted to decrease the federally subsidized unemployment benefits under the *CARES Act* by $400 per week).

Their expressed rationale was that the $600 per week funded unemployment benefits contributed to people not wanting to return to work.[215]

Okay, help me to understand! Why should a person laid-off from a low-paid job (with no health insurance offered) who is especially vulnerable to Covid-19, or has an immunocompromised family member at high risk of death from Covid-19, want to return to that job and risk the lives of everyone in their household?

Inequity is the root cause of the disproportionate effect of Covid-19 on Black and Brown people, and this absolutely has to change before the *next* pandemic.

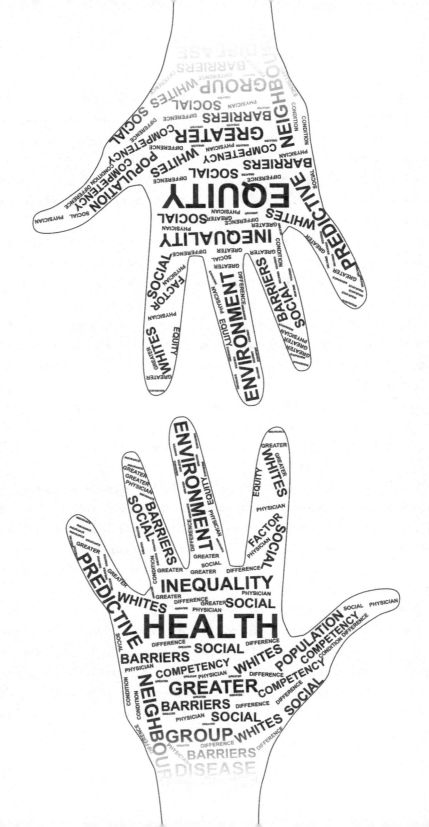

CHAPTER 15

Δ

HEALTH JUSTICE AND EQUITY ADVOCACY: ROLE OF FAITH LEADERS, NONPROFITS, AND COMMUNITY SOCIAL AND CIVIC GROUPS

Psalm 82:3 commands us to "give justice to the poor and the orphan; uphold the rights of the oppressed and the destitute" (*Holy Bible*, New Living Translation).

Collaboration is Essential

As community and faith-based leaders (regardless of profession), we are called to lead in a manner that considers the lives of those among us who are less fortunate. Moreover, in developing strategies and action plans to meet the needs of our community members, we would be remiss to neglect the voices of our marginalized populations.

Community in conjunction with faith-based organizations must play a role in promoting equitable access to worthwhile, affordable care. In some cases, this can mean taking steps to bring the care to the community. Mark 9:35 says, "If anyone would be first, he must be last of all and servant of all" (*The Holy Bible*, English Standard Version).

We must work together to ensure that the members of our communities have the necessary tools and resources to promote mental and physical health and wellness. Our programs must be housed at the churches, recreation centers, or community buildings where our community lives, learns, worships, works, and plays.

The creation of Equity Clinics for Covid vaccinations is a prime example of how we must deploy resources. We have scheduled vaccine clinics within the community that are easily accessible, and we are working together to provide transportation.

Meanwhile, we must also recognize that the days of "we build it, and they will come" are over. This means that we must not do anything to our community members without our community members.

In other words, we must enlist them in the planning process. They deserve a "seat at the table," and we must become advocates for their voices to be heard and incorporated. This will bring us toward the ultimate goal of eliminating health disparities along with providing quality, equitable care to *everyone*!

However, the above-described goals cannot be accomplished in a silo; we must rely on the involvement of community partners. One strategy to foster a collaborative partnership with community members is to train barbers, beauticians, pastors, other clergy, and other influential community members to be both physical and mental health advocates.

The church is the center of the African American community. This is where we go for refuge, hope, and direction. Likewise, we trust the elders of our congregations and community members customarily confide in these elder members, even when not willing to confide in anyone else.

Despite numerous nonprofit organizations, including spiritually oriented nonprofits with a focus on the same population demographic, there is all too often a lack of pooling the existing resources and efforts. The result is a weak and fractured approach to aiding that population.

We have multiple nonprofits touching the same demographics of people, yet we are not pooling our resources and efforts. We tend to be resource-rich yet connectivity-poor.

The profit margin cannot become more important than the mission. There has to be a nice mellow rhythm between the two. We should focus on practicing servant leadership principles. A servant leader offers an inclusive vision, listens carefully to others, persuades through reason, and heals divisions while building community.

Notably, instead of being self-serving, we in leadership positions must see ourselves as servants of the community in order to aid that community. In other words, an *effective* leader must act as a "servant leader."

An effective "servant leader" is a person who has an inclusive vision, listens carefully to others, persuades through reasoning, and heals divisions while also building community.

What is Health Justice?

In terms of addressing the SDoH and other related issues, health justice means creating equity. It is crucial to understand that this cannot be accomplished in a silo but instead requires learning from one another, sharing best practices, and good old-fashioned collaboration.

Fostered in a patient/client-centered approach, Health Care Systems (HCSs), Public Health Systems (PHSs), and organizations designated as Community Partners must collaboratively address the inequities encountered in marginalized communities.

After all, our communities' abilities to thrive are dependent upon healthy people living in healthy communities. Therefore, for those working to advance healthcare system reforms, we must focus on the patient perspective and the impact that the reforms we embrace have on their lived experiences.

To address the SDoH and eliminate the identified inequities, we must include an intentional focus to our social justice advocacy for health equity along with criminal justice and education justice. In reality, health justice matters for health equity; health justice cultivates health equity.

Health justice means that marginalized and vulnerable populations need to be respected in our society, and health insurance needs to be viewed as a *right* rather than a *privilege*.

To achieve health justice, the structural barriers leading to health inequity for marginalized communities need to be dismantled. Acquiring data that can be measured regarding the disparities confronting marginalized communities is also vital.

What is measured gets addressed in the healthcare policy and advocacy realm. Therefore, it is essential to understand what data is available, access it, and then ask the appropriate questions to drive change.

Engage public health students and city and county epidemiologists to focus more on the health-related conditions disproportionally impacting marginalized populations and thus, potentially help everyone, not just the privileged, to have an equitable opportunity to become healthier.

According to Dr. Dwayne Proctor, Director and Senior Advisor at the Robert Wood Foundation, "Health disparities not only affect the day-to-day experiences of individuals but also threatens the prosperity and well-being of entire communities."[216]

> *Most of all, please understand. Health justice is not an "Us against Them" problem, but instead our problem.*

Most of all, please understand. Health justice is not an "Us against Them" problem, but instead *our* problem. Therefore, we must work together and focus on providing each person with what they need, at the right time and in the right place. We all have skin in this game—so let's move forward with that in mind!

CHAPTER 16

Δ

ADVOCATING FOR BETTER HEALTHCARE
FOR YOURSELF

This will sound cliché, but it is true. Your body is the temple of your soul. Therefore, you need to take care of your body, and that includes advocating for better healthcare for yourself and being an engaged and active partner to your health care professionals.

It also means that if you are a US citizen and not a person of color, it is incumbent upon you to act as an "ally" in advocating for better healthcare for people of color.

As the Covid-19 pandemic has revealed (and continues to reveal), we need to work together to improve public health for *everyone*.

Not just for white people or "owning-class" people. The inequities based on class and "race" in the US are pervasive and systemic. Likewise, these inequities pervade the US health system—and thus disproportionately burden Black and Brown people.

What Can You Do?

We must educate ourselves so that we can be empowered to transform our current state of reality. We must not allow others who hold either *overt* or *covert* biases and prejudices to present a distorted perception of our existence.

Take Action by Speaking Up

When we visit our healthcare providers, we must hold them accountable; we must demand the same high-quality treatment, respect, and cultural sensitivity that is afforded to others not of our gender, "race," or socioeconomic status—and/or who have grand levels of education; greater community and social stability; and more comprehensive health insurance coverage.

When we are not treated equitably, we must talk to the executive leaders of the health care facilities that we frequent about the problems fostering inequity in healthcare. The truth is that we must become comfortable with making others uncomfortable.

Familiarize Yourself with Services and Resources

Familiarize yourself with the culturally relevant community services and resources that are available to you, such as clinical therapists of color or faith-based therapists of color in your area.

You can accomplish this by reaching out to local community agencies, such as your Urban Leagues and other civic groups. You can conduct Google searches for minority clinicians in your area.

Take time to visit the website of your insurance plan, where you can find names and oftentimes photos. You can also go to the hospital website to view a list of clinicians with photos. Word of mouth is always great. Talk with friends, colleagues, and church members.

Read Google and Yelp reviews on health care providers. There is a wealth of information at your fingertips, so please take the time to conduct your research.

Above all, you *need* to believe that you deserve worthwhile healthcare. This means not accepting the *status quo* of an inferior standard of care, assuming you did something to deserve it, or thinking that the state of your healthcare actually does not matter all that much.

Do Not Become Frustrated and Just Give Up

Please do not become frustrated and decide, "I'm just not going to go back." This only leads to reduced health outcomes such as cancer progression moving from treatable to terminal, diabetes leading to amputation of limbs, hypertension ending in a stroke, heart attack, or death.

Your health concerns will not correct themselves; they will probably worsen. Annual preventive visits, such as well visit health physicals, are vital to lessen the likelihood of developing a chronic health disorder in the first place!

Become an Educated Consumer Who Can Make Good Decisions

Do not let a prior negative encounter deter you from continuing your health and wellness journey—but realize that you will need to become an educated consumer to make the best decisions for your health and medical care.

Yes, you will need to become educated about seeking out and obtaining quality healthcare to increase the likelihood that you will get it!

Being an educated consumer includes understanding how to determine if your physician(s) and other healthcare providers have a good reputation for providing their healthcare services; is practicing with a current clinical license, has a reasonable level of experience as a healthcare clinician; and is considered "culturally-competent" with exemplary bedside manner.

If any of these things are not true, you may need to attempt to find a different clinician in whom to entrust your care!

Take the Required Steps Toward Living the Healthiest Lifestyle Possible for You

You need to live a lifestyle that will promote your health and wellness. This is necessary so that you can prevent developing an avoidable chronic health condition— or avoid *worsening* an already-present chronic health condition.

The two lifestyle factors most associated with worsened health and well-being are smoking and having a Body Mass Index (BMI) correlated to clinical obesity. Meanwhile, substance use disorders (*e.g.,* alcohol and/or drugs) can negatively impact brain function leading to bad decisions and permanent harm to interpersonal relationships, which can result in a worsened quality of life.

In addition, you need to be careful not to fall for "fad" diets, treatments, or pills. Many unscrupulous businesses target Black and Brown people with "fad" health-boosters that cost a lot of money but deliver nothing *and* can even worsen health. There are reliable online health information sources such as the Mayo Clinic's website (and other teaching hospital websites).

In terms of boosting your immune system so that you can better fight infections, there are things you can do. The most important is to ensure that you are getting the Recommended Daily Allowance (RDA) of all vitamins and minerals.

The best way to do this is by consuming a balanced daily diet. If you cannot do this, speak with your PCP about recommendations for taking a daily multivitamin.

Other ways to boost your immunity are to get enough nightly sleep, complete at least fifteen minutes of daily exercise, and manage emotional stress and anxiety. Practicing meditation, yoga, or another relaxation technique daily can aid you in reducing anxiety.

If you subscribe to Netflix, Amazon Prime, or Hulu, they have videos included in your subscription that you can stream in the comfort of your home.

The National Center for Complementary and Integrative Health website describes various research articles concluding the benefits of meditation and relaxation techniques for the following health issues: pain, high blood pressure, irritable bowel syndrome, ulcerative colitis, anxiety/depression/insomnia, smoking cessation, and other health-impacting conditions.[217]

State Boards of Registration in Medicine

Nearly every state in the US has a Board of Registration in Medicine that oversees physician licensure. While every state in the US requires that actively practicing physicians be licensed, the requirements can differ between states.[218]

Most states enable online public searching by physician's name to learn the following: 1) whether that physician has an active license to practice medicine, 2) the specialty field in which that physician is licensed, 3) when (and where) that physician graduated from medical school, 4) the name of the medical school attended, and 5) whether any malpractice lawsuits were filed against that physician.

Therefore, it makes sense to search for information about any physician providing you care, especially if you are told by your Primary Care Physician (PCP) that you need to schedule an appointment with a specialist physician.

Suppose the physician from whom you are seeking information accepts Medicare or Medicaid insurance. In that case, much of the same information available in most online Board of Registration in Medicine databases is available via an online search in the Medicare.gov website called "Physician Compare."[219]

Informed Consent Forms

My advice is to never sign an *Informed Consent* form from a healthcare provider without reading it. If you do not understand the form, have someone you trust explain it to you.

If your native language is not English (and you have Limited English Proficiency [LEP]), request the *Informed Consent* form be provided in your native language or insist on an interpreter to translate it, but do not let the physician simply explain it to you and then sign it.

As someone having LEP, you have specific rights as a patient under Executive Order 13166 of Title VI of the federal 1964 *Civil Rights Act* as well as Section 1557 of the *Affordable Care Act* (ACA).

Therefore, any healthcare facility that receives federal financial assistance (through the DHSS) is required to provide language interpreter services for someone who needs such services.[220]

The truth is that you will need to be your own advocate, so if you feel uncomfortable questioning your physician or provider about a new diagnosis or

> *The truth is that you will need to be your own advocate, so if you feel uncomfortable questioning your physician or provider about a new diagnosis or treatment plan, it is best to bring someone you trust with you to the medical appointment.*

treatment plan, it is best to bring someone you trust with you to the medical appointment.

That trusted person's presence may be all that is needed to give you the courage to actively engage with your physician and acquire the appropriate healthcare services and treatment plans!

No one will care more about you than you, so engage, advocate, make wise lifestyle choices that impact your health, and follow through on all health-related matters.

CHAPTER 17

Δ

WHAT WHITE PEOPLE CAN DO AS ALLIES TO END HEALTH-IMPACTING INEQUITIES

This chapter is aimed at the white readers. Everyone needs allies, and you are to be commended for caring enough to read this book to its last chapter. However, recognizing the inequities faced by people of color in terms of healthcare is not enough. You need to take action.

If you have never read an article or book on anti-racism aimed at white people, my advice is to read one of the books recommended in the New York Magazine article on June 5, 2020, "Anti-Racist Books Recommended by Educators and Activists."

This article particularly commends the book, *How to Be an Antiracist* by Ibram X. Kendi.[221] Or attend a workshop or class focused on increasing your "cultural competence/sensitivity."

To better understand the pervasive way oppression works, you may benefit from reading the book written by Albert Memmi in 1957 titled *The Colonizer and The Colonized*. While this French-Algerian author never lived in the US, the book examines the diverse ways institutionalized oppression impacts both the oppressor and oppressed in ways that disable both from living freely.

Challenge the prejudiced opinions of colleagues and others in your workplace expressed about people of color and report any discriminatory speech or actions toward employees of color you witness to entities legally required to act (*e.g.,* your employer's Human Resources Department or the nearest office to you of the US Equal Employment Opportunity Commission [*EEOC*]).

If you can afford it, donate financially to nonprofit organizations that benefit low-income residents of Black and Brown communities.

You can also donate to the local and state political campaigns of a person of color running for office to build the presence of people of color in the political arena who are proponents of policies decreasing inequities disproportionately faced by people of color.

If you like to retail shop, buy more often from retail businesses owned by African American, Latinx, Asian, and Native American people.

The reality is that most companies owned by people of color face more financial and legal obstacles to growth than white-owned businesses, so your patronage may enable a struggling business to turn a profit.

Join groups focused on reducing healthcare disparities affecting people of color and listen to understand and not just to respond (rather than just *talk)* to the people of color in the group.

Of course, an enormous way you can take action as an "ally" is by voting for political candidates at the local, state, and federal levels that want—and have shown evidence of the political will by their voting record—to dismantle structural racism in the US.

I say all of that to say this, your action (and inaction) in working against inequities in our society do matter.

Ida B. Wells-Barnett (a founding member of the *National Association for the Advancement of Colored People* [*NAACP*], and a journalist, educator, and early leader in the Civil Rights Movement) said: "One had better die fighting against injustice than die like a dog or rat in a trap."

I say all of that to say this, your action (and inaction) in working against inequities in our society do matter. We need to continue to resist injustice! But for the grace of God, it could be you!

PART IV

QUESTIONS TO PROMOTE YOUR THOUGHT, KNOWLEDGE, AND SELF-AWARENESS

1. How has the Covid-19 pandemic affected your life (or anyone in your family or network of friends)? [Choose no more than five ways to describe.]

_____

_____

_____

_____

_____

_____

2. If you were aware before reading this book that people of color were more likely to become very ill or die from Covid19, how does this make you feel?

_____

_____

_____

_____

_____

_____

3. Has religion or spirituality helped or hindered you in your life? How has this helped or hindered your life? [Choose no more than four ways to describe.]

_____

_____

_____

_____

_____

_____

4. Who are five faith leaders _or_ leaders of nonprofit or community-based organizations that you feel are role models or inspirations for you? Why?

_____

_____

_____

_____

_____

_____

5. What are five ways that you have taken action since you became an adult to take care of your body and overall health?

_____

_____

_____

_____

_____

6. Are your usual lifestyle and daily life boosting or harming your health? And how do you feel they boost or worsen your *mental* health?

_____

_____

_____

_____

_____

7. Do you eat a balanced diet, get enough sleep, manage your stress level, and get enough weekly exercise? What do you feel that you still need to do to take better care of your health?

_____

_____

_____

_____

_____

8. What keeps you from taking actions that you know would improve your overall health and well-being? If you do not feel that any action by you would improve your overall health and well-being, why do you feel this way?

_____

_____

_____

_____

_____

9. What organizations or groups working to improve the lives of people of color do you admire? Why?

_____

_____

_____

_____

_____

10. What actions can you take to change the *status quo* in terms of discrimination and inequities faced by people of color in the US?

_____

_____

_____

_____

_____

CONCLUSION

An individual's health outcome is partially determined by how well one takes care of himself/herself; it is also determined by the SDoH (*e.g.*, socioeconomic status). Therefore, we all must be able to live in environments that are conducive to good health.

Living conditions are "influencers" on our health. Indeed, the neighborhood in which you live can reduce your life expectancy by up to thirty years. Therefore, your zip code (rather than your genes) is the greatest predictor of your life expectancy. This is mind-blowing and absolutely unacceptable!

Perhaps you are familiar with the following saying attributable to Confucius (a Chinese philosopher who lived in the sixth Century BC) "If you give a man a fish, he will eat for a day, but if you teach him to fish, he will eat for a lifetime."

Or will he? Although this belief has been fundamental to public policy for US citizens over the past 100 years, this belief does not consider equity and systemic or institutionalized racism.

The erroneous assumption is that each person can equally afford the fishing lesson, and the equipment and supplies necessary to *fish* at all.

Does the fisherman have access to a pond that is not polluted? Does the pond actually have enough fish to feed him and his family on a daily basis? Does he have any disabilities that would prevent him from being able to fish?

Does he live in a warm climate where the pond does not freeze over, and if he doesn't, does he have the tools necessary for ice fishing?

I think you get the gist of where I am going with this. Policymakers must aid disadvantaged communities to be able to overcome the many inequities contributing to worsened health!

We must begin to meet patients where they are, and when it comes to the delivery of healthcare. There is a misconception that people are poor because they made bad decisions when, in actuality, they are making "tough" decisions because of poverty.

This is the truth. Oppressed populations are not oppressing themselves; they are not lazy. They do need the "system" to have compassion and create equitable practices. For all travelers on the road, the distance may be the same between Point A to Point B.

However, the obstacles presented along the way are vastly different for some groups of people in the US than others, which is *inequity*.

Allison Massari stated the following in response to an interview question: "compassion heals the places that medicine cannot touch."[222] This is a statement that I am sharing with you because it has a particular meaning for me.

In my perspective, compassion and equity deeply intertwine. When we think and operate in the healthcare realm in the "space" of compassion, we move from delivering *transactional* care to *transformational* care. Compassion creates equity!

Simply stated, the right cure requires the right diagnosis. The steps necessary for our society to achieve this goal involve setting a goal of *equity* in healthcare.

We must find ways to effectively move forward, enable the most vulnerable in our society to find their voice and be heard and engage public health students as well as public health professionals to increase knowledge and awareness of the SDoH that disproportionally impact Black and Brown communities.

It is important to always remember that "To whom much is given, much shall be required" (Luke 12:48, *Aramaic Bible* in Plain English). We are blessed to be a blessing to others, and as a healthcare professional, I stand firmly on this principle, which is yet another reason I've created this body of work.

Indeed, I believe that it is incumbent upon community leaders and healthcare professionals alike to implement policies, procedures, and initiatives that foster equity and improve the health of those who entrust their lives to us.

Systemic racism and bigoted attitudes toward people of color underpin the disparities in health across the United States between white people and people of color.

While public health data clearly shows these disparities in graphs revealing the burden of chronic health conditions among Black and Brown children and adults, the reasons for the discrepancies are not revealed by such graphs. Nor do these graphs *explain* the worse medical care outcomes and lower life expectancy for people of color compared to the white people in this nation.

Despite growing recognition of the impact of the social determinants of health on overall health and well-being, the impact of institutionalized racism on these social determinants remains mostly unacknowledged in the public health and medical research arenas.

As you are now well aware from reading this book, the social determinants of health include every aspect of daily life from birth to death. Eating, holding a job, keeping a roof over one's head, and accessing affordable quality healthcare when needed all impact overall health across the continuum of life.

A person born into impoverishment is more prone to develop chronic health disorders over time than someone not growing up below the poverty level.

Yet, understanding this reality does not actually answer the question, "Why?" which is one of the primary reasons this book was written. That answer is critical to understanding why impoverished people of color are vastly more likely than impoverished white people to develop chronic health problems with a concomitant to elevated risk for premature death.

Over the past forty years, an increasing number of public health research studies have repeatedly revealed that living in poverty is linked to worsened overall health and a raised mortality rate. Low educational attainment has also been associated with worsened overall health over the lifespan. Ditto for lack of health insurance or lack of access to preventive healthcare services.

When these social determinants are viewed not individually but as a combined force greater than the sum of the diverse parts, the tremendous impact of systemic racism on health in the US is obvious.

Such research has also repeatedly shown that white US residents *as a population* are more likely to have better healthcare outcomes than African American, Latinx, and Native American residents.

Problematically, studying each social determinant and its effect on people of color in the US does not really allow for recognition of racism as the underlying reason.

Moreover, most of these study findings have been published by white public health and medical researchers who—while predominantly well-meaning in choosing to study the impact of the social determinants of health— are not especially focused on dismantling systemic racism.

Here is the "ah-ha" moment! When these social determinants are viewed *not* individually but as a combined force greater than the sum of the diverse parts, the tremendous impact of systemic racism on health in the US is obvious.

In other words, it is the *societal inequities* that lead to inequity in terms of overall health status and quality of life disadvantage of US residents who are Black and Brown, and regardless of socioeconomic status, educational attainment, or employment role.

In a metaphor embodied in the Racial Equity Institute's report, "The Groundwater Approach: Building a Practical Understanding of Structural Racism,"[223] structural racism is embedded in the groundwater of US society.

By using the *groundwater* metaphor, the reader is enabled to better grasp how the diverse structures of our society ensure the persistence of racial inequity.

As the Racial Equity Institute's website notes, "The premise for the metaphor is as follows: racial inequity looks the same across systems; socioeconomic difference does not explain the racial inequity; and inequities are caused by systems, regardless of people's culture or behavior."[224]

This free, downloadable report was written while the Covid-19 pandemic has been raging across the US, with a disproportionately high rate of infection and death occurring among people of color across this country.

The current Covid-19 pandemic has shined an undeniable spotlight on the underlying societal factors that have led to the larger Covid-19 fatality rate for people of color in the US as measured alongside the white population.

No longer can anyone in the US reasonably argue that societal factors are unimportant as factors contributing to health outcomes. We all know otherwise due to this coronavirus pandemic.

Within its four separate but related parts, this book introduced you to the diverse societal determinants of health and well-being and the disparities faced by people of color concerning each of these determinants.

However, included in this book were not only the usual determinants of healthcare outcomes but the adverse impact of the lack of Black and Brown healthcare clinicians in the US, as well as the widespread racist assumptions of some healthcare professionals.

Additionally, an overview of the historical mistreatment of people of color by the US health system *and* the higher rate of imprisonment of Black and Brown people were included as factors impacting overall health status.

The Argument for Reparations

In the past decade, the commencement of a discussion as to whether reparations are owed to people of color in the US has occurred. This argument for reparations has a historical foundation.

Such a discussion happened at the formal end of the apartheid system in South Africa, with the subsequent establishment of a national Truth and Reconciliation Commission (TRC) that developed federal policy recommendations in 1998, resulting in recognition of the need for reparations and an implementation plan.[225]

While the idea of reparations is often dismissed in the US as impossible due to an assumption that a monetary amount to each person of color would be the basis of such reparations, this dismissal ignores the ongoing health impact on people of color of systemic racism.

Instead of reparation dollars provided to a particular person of color, my belief is that this money is owed to entire communities could take the form of free medical school education, a greater proportion of federal education dollars allotted to schools in Black and Brown neighborhoods, investment in Historically Black Colleges and Universities (HBCUs), federal and state grants for Black and Brown small businesses, and other financial assistance to contribute to society-wide *equality* and economic development.

Identifying and addressing inequities is essential, but promoting *equality* remains the underlying goal. As this book has demonstrated, the impact of the social determinants of health has been worsened health and shortened lifespans for people of color in the US.

One way you can resist the systemic racism underpinning healthcare-related disparities is to live the healthiest lifestyle that you can. However, dismantling the society-wide systemic racism in the US needs to occur for nationwide public health *for all* to exist.

As the Covid-19 pandemic has continued to show, inclusive of the vaccine "roll-out," our health and well-being, are essential to enabling better health status across the entire population.

If you have acquired nothing else from reading this book, take *action* to take care of your mind, body, spirit, and your physical health. And counterattack the systemic oppression of Black and Brown people. Yes, it takes a village!

ACKNOWLEDGMENTS

Frist and foremost, I would like to give honor and praise to God because I never would have made it without Him! He is my strength, my salvation, and my redeemer, and I am grateful for His grace, mercy, and favor.

I would like to thank my village for believing in me and encouraging me to complete this project over the past three years. My sister, friend, and soror, Dr. Teresa Myers (the author of my forward), holds my deepest gratitude for her insight and guidance throughout my career as a healthcare leader.

You poured into me and put me on the track of utterly understanding the fundamental foundation and necessity of health equity.

I would like to express my appreciation to Darren Palmer and the phenomenal team at Self Publish -N- 30 Days for the editing, proofreading, cover design, and publication of this book.

I jokingly referred to Darren as "Bishop" because, during our weekly consultation calls, he was sure to give what we in the Black church call a "word," and he backed it with scripture for me to meditate on until our next call. Darren, you truly encouraged my soul when I most needed it.

In addition, I would like to thank my soror and line sister, Dr. Jennifer Ross, for proofreading my manuscript and providing me with her feedback, insight, and wisdom.

Thank you to my godbrother and published author, Dr. Eric Johnson, for your insight and willingness to proofread my manuscript.

Thank you, MariHelyn Horrigan, LPN, for lighting the fire inside me I needed to finally put pen to paper and begin this journey. You are a firecracker and a genuine ally for the Black and Brown community. I am enamored by your commitment to eradicating SDoH.

To Dr. Patrick J. Fernicola, who many years ago showed me through his actions what it meant to be a servant leader. Over the past two decades, I have done my best to emulate the qualities you so genuinely display.

I'd also like to thank a couple of Emergency Department nurses that I met one evening while having a dinner meeting to discuss health equity with State

Representative of the 49th District of the Ohio House of Representatives Tom West;- Jamie Hill, RN, and Scott Rice, RN.

We are from different worlds with different world views; however, we had a thought-provoking conversation around political viewpoints, health care delivery in general, and, of course, health justice.

Scott asked me the title of my book (which originally was far too wordy and ambiguous). When I told him, he instantly said it was "too long." We brainstormed together and landed on the current title, and he said, "If I saw that title, it would draw me to read it!" I agreed, and here we are (See, I told you I was going to acknowledge you).

I am grateful to my aunt, Kimberly Jenkins-Snodgrass, who is also a published author and my uncle Kevin Snodgrass, for believing in me and encouraging me to "birth this book."

I would like to thank my daddy in Heaven, Keith D. Snodgrass Sr., for his continual affirmation of the endless possibilities for my life. He taught me as a little girl that I have a voice and to never let anyone stunt my growth by silencing me.

In his own way, he taught me that my voice counts and that I must make space for myself at tables because I not only deserve to be there, but I deserve to be included in the conversation.

His love taught me to find comfort in my discomfort, and it instilled a passion for helping others the way my village has helped me.

My mother, Shirley A. Lewis, who spent the majority of her life caring for others, you are a true inspiration and a strong woman that has supported me in ways that only a mother could.

My brother, Keith D. Snodgrass Jr., LSW, who shares my passion for serving oppressed populations and talked with me about the premise for this book, the insight you shared gave me the strength to see this project through.

Then there is my son, Tommie "TJ" Harris III, whose unconditional love pushed me to the finish line.

I'd be remiss not to thank Tim Bushner for your encouragement, love and support. For always telling me what I needed to hear and not necessarily what I wanted to hear. For keeping me accountable to my milestones even when I felt like throwing in the towel. Tough love is definitely necessary, and I am grateful for yours.

I cannot possibly name everyone in my village that has played a part but please know I am humbled by your support, transparency, enthusiasm, encouragement, and love.

Reader, I address you last. Thank you for taking the first step toward health equality by picking up this book. The disparities faced in our country are much bigger than the book in your hand, but it is my hope that in reading this, you will be better equipped to go out into the world and make positive change.

The first step to solving any problem is acknowledging that it exists, so thank you for taking the first step by mediating on this issue with me.

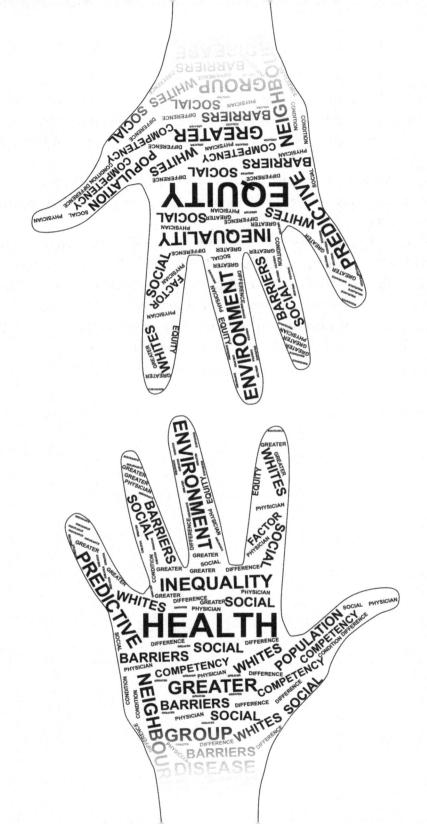

REFERENCES

1 Healthy People 2020. Framework. *The Vision, Mission, and Goals of Healthy People* 2020. https://www.healthypeople.gov/sites/default/files/HP2020Framework.pdf

2 National Public Radio (NPR). *Code Switch.* (January 14, 2014). *The Code Switch Podcast*: Making the Case that Discrimination is Bad for Your Health. Wepage: https://www.npr.org/sections/codeswitch/2018/01/14/577664626/making-the-case-that-discrimination-is-bad-for-your-health

3 Centers for Disease Control and Prevention. (2020). National Diabetes Statistics Report 2020: Estimates of Diabetes and Its Burden in the United States. [Publication No.: CS 314227-A]. Webpage: https://www.cdc.gov/diabetes/pdfs/data/statistics/national-diabetes-statistics-report.pdf

4 Asthma and Allergy Foundation of America (AAFA). (2005) Ethnic Disparities in the Burden and Treatment of Asthma.Webpage: https://www.aafa.org/media/1633/ethnic-disparities-burden-treatment-asthma-report.pdf

5 Niv N, Pham R, and Hser YI. (2009). Racial and ethnic differences in substance abuse service needs, utilization, and outcomes in California. *Psychiatr Services* 60(10): 1350-1356. Webpage: https://www.ncbi.nlm.nih.gov/pmc/articles/PMC2821670/

6 Wilkerson, Isabel. (2011). *The Warmth of Other Suns.* Random House: NY.

7 Miriam-Webster Dictionary. Legal Definition – Redlining. Webpage: https://www.merriam-webster.com/legal/redlining

8 Rothstein, Richard. (2017). The Color of Law. W.W. Norton & Co: NY.

9 The Urban Institute. (February 21, 2020). Breaking Down the Black-White Homeownership Gap. Webpage: https://www.urban.org/urban-wire/breaking-down-black-white-homeownership-gap

10 American Cancer Society. *Cancer Facts and Figures for African Americans*, 2019-2020. Webpage: https://www.cancer.org/content/dam/cancer-org/

research/cancer-facts-and-statistics/cancer-facts-and-figures-for-african-americans/cancer-facts-and-figures-for-african-americans-2019-2021.pdf

[11] National Cancer Institute, Division of Cancer Epidemiology and Genetics. Webpage: https://dceg.cancer.gov/research/what-we-study/drinking-water-contaminants

[12] Kirtane K, and Lee SJ. (2017). Racial and ethnic disparities in hematologic malignancies. *Blood* 130(15): 1699-1705. Webpage: https://www.ncbi.nlm.nih.gov/pmc/articles/PMC5639484/

[13] Harr, Jonathan. (1996). *A Civil Action*. Random House: NY.

[14] Hanna-Attisha, Mona. (2018). *What the Eyes Don't See*. Penguin Random House: NY.

[15] US Dept. of Housing and Urban Development (HUD). *Public Housing*. Webpage: https://www.hud.gov/program_offices/public_indian_housing/programs/ph#:~:text=Public%20housing%20comes%20in%20all,managed%20by%20some%203300%20PHAs.

[16] Kaiser Family Foundation (KFF). (2018). Poverty Rate by Race/Ethnicity. Webpage: https://www.kff.org/other/state-indicator/poverty-rate-by-raceethnicity/?currentTimeframe=0&sortModel=%7B%22colId%22:%22Location%22,%22sort%22:%22asc%22%7D

[17] US Dept. of Housing and Urban Development (HUD). US Housing Market Conditions Summary; Public Housing: Image versus Facts. Webpage: https://www.huduser.gov/periodicals/ushmc/spring95/spring95.html#:~:text=Forty%2Deight%20percent%20of%20public,percent%20of%20all%20renter%20households.

[18] Public Broadcasting System (PBS), KQED. Fillmore Timeline: 1860-2001. Webpage: https://www.pbs.org/kqed/fillmore/learning/time.html

[19] Pew Research Center. (May 22, 2018). What Unites and Divides Urban, Suburban, and Rural Communities; 5. Americans' satisfaction with and attachment to

their communities. Webpage: https://www.pewsocialtrends.org/2018/05/22/americans-satisfaction-with-and-attachment-to-their-communities/

20 Lewis J, Hoover J, and MacKenzie D. (2017). Mining and Environmental Health Disparities in Native American Communities. *Current Environmental Health Reports* 4(2): 130-141. Webpage: https://www.ncbi.nlm.nih.gov/pmc/articles/PMC5429369/

21 Szentpetery SE, Forno E, Canino G, and Celedón JC. (2016). Asthma in Puerto Ricans: Lessons from a high-risk population. *J Allergy Clin Immunol.* 138(6):1556-1558. Webpage: https://www.ncbi.nlm.nih.gov/pmc/articles/PMC5189666/

22 IndexMundi.com. Puerto Rico - Urban population (% of total population). Webpage: https://www.indexmundi.com/facts/puerto-rico/indicator/SP.URB.TOTL.IN.ZS

23 United States Courts. Supreme Court Landmarks: History – Brown v. Board of Education Re-enactment. Webpage: https://www.uscourts.gov/educational-resources/educational-activities/history-brown-v-board-education-re-enactment

24 Menand, Louis. (January 13, 2020). The Changing Meaning of Affirmative Action. *The New Yorker* Webpage: https://www.newyorker.com/magazine/2020/01/20/have-we-outgrown-the-need-for-affirmative-action

25 American Association for Access, Equity and Diversity (AAAED). More History of Affirmative Action Policies from the 1960s. Webpage: https://www.aaaed.org/aaaed/History_of_Affirmative_Action.asp

26 US National Center for Education Statistics (NCES). (Last Updated: May 2020). Public High School Graduation Rates. Webpage: https://nces.ed.gov/programs/coe/indicator_coi.asp

27 Camera L. (March 23, 2016). The College Graduation Gap Is Still Growing. *US News and World Report* Web-

page: https://www.usnews.com/news/blogs/data-mine/2016/03/23/study-college-graduation-gap-between-blacks-whites-still-growing

28 US National Center for Education Statistics (NCES). Fast Facts: Race/Ethnicity of College Faculty. Webpage: https://nces.ed.gov/fastfacts/display.asp?id=61

29 National Education Association (NEA). Charter Schools 101. Webpage: http://www.nea.org/home/60831.htm

30 Pennsylvania State Education Association (PSEA). What Has Betsy DeVos Done? Webpage: https://www.psea.org/issues-action/key-issues/betsy-devos-timeline/

31 Green EL. (June 28, 2019). DeVos Repeals Obama-Era Rule Cracking Down on For-Profit Colleges. *New York Times* Webpage: https://www.nytimes.com/2019/06/28/us/politics/betsy-devos-for-profit-colleges.html

32 Northern Arizona University. American Indian School Dropouts and Pushouts. Webpage: https://jan.ucc.nau.edu/~jar/AIE/Dropouts.html

33 Association of American Medical Colleges (AAMC). Diversity in Medicine: Facts and Figures 2019. Webpage: https://www.aamc.org/data-reports/workforce/interactive-data/figure-18-percentage-all-active-physicians-race/ethnicity-2018

34 Chen FM, Fryer GE, Phillips RL, et al. (2005). Patients' Beliefs About Racism, Preferences for Physician Race, and Satisfaction With Care. *Annals of Family Medicine* 3(2): 138-143. Webpage: https://www.annfammed.org/content/3/2/138.full?maxtoshow=&hits=20&RESULTFORMAT=&searchid=1&FIRSTINDEX=260&displaysectionid=Original+Research&resourcetype=HWCIT

35 Louie, P. and Wilkes Rima. (April 2018). Representations of race and skin tone in medical textbook imagery. *Social Science & Medicine*, 202, 38-42. https://doi.org/10.1016/j.socscimed.2018.02.023.

[36] Hoffman, K. M., Trawalter, S., Axt, J. R., & Oliver, M. N. (April 4, 2016). Racial bias in pain assessment and treatment recommendations, and false beliefs about biological differences between blacks and whites. *Proceedings of the National Academy of Sciences,* 113(16), 4296–4301. Webpage: https://www.ncbi.nlm.nih.gov/pmc/articles/PMC4843483/

[37] Campbell S. (February 2018). Research Brief – Racial Disparities in the Direct Care Workforce: Spotlight on Black/African American Workers. PHI International Webpage: https://phinational.org/wp-content/uploads/2018/02/Black-Direct-Care-Workers-PHI-2018.pdf

[38] US Bureau of Labor Statistics. (February 13, 2019). TED: The Economics Daily. Rising educational attainment among Blacks or African Americans in the labor force, 1992 to 2018. Webpage: https://www.bls.gov/opub/ted/2019/rising-educational-attainment-among-blacks-or-african-americans-in-the-labor-force-1992-to-2018.htm

[39] Pew Research Center. (July 1, 2016). Racial, gender wage gaps persist in U.S. despite some progress. Webpage: https://www.pewresearch.org/fact-tank/2016/07/01/racial-gender-wage-gaps-persist-in-u-s-despite-some-progress/

[40] National Partnership for Women and Families. (March 2020). Quantifying America's Gender Wage Gap by Race/Ethnicity. Webpage: https://www.nationalpartnership.org/our-work/resources/economic-justice/fair-pay/quantifying-americas-gender-wage-gap.pdf

[41] Rogers TN. (June 12, 2020). There are 615 billionaires in the United States, and only 6 of them are Black. Business Insider Webpage: https://www.businessinsider.com/black-billionaires-in-the-united-states-2020-2

[42] United Way of New Jersey. Meet ALICE. Webpage: https://www.unitedforalice.org/

[43] Rebel Interactive Group. United Way ALICE Poverty Simulator. https://rebelinteractivegroup.com/united-way-alice-poverty-simulator/

44 US Federal Highway Administration. (2014). NHTS Brief: Mobility Challenges for Households in Poverty. Webpage: https://nhts.ornl.gov/briefs/PovertyBrief.pdf

45 The National Archives (of the UK). Victorian Railways. Webpage: https://www.nationalarchives.gov.uk/education/resources/victorian-railways/

46 CNBC News. (May 26, 2020). Amtrak needs $1.5 billion bailout, prepares to cut up to 20% of workforce. Webpage: https://www.cnbc.com/2020/05/27/amtrak-needs-bailout-plans-to-cut-up-to-20-percent-of-workforce.html

47 CNBC News. (May 9, 2018). Congress eases rules against racial discrimination in the auto loan market. Webpage: https://www.cnbc.com/2018/05/09/congress-eases-rules-against-racial-discrimination-in-the-auto-loan-market.html

48 Satia JA. (2009). Diet-related disparities: understanding the problem and accelerating solutions. *J Am Diet Assoc*. 109(4): 610-615. Webpage: https://www.ncbi.nlm.nih.gov/pmc/articles/PMC2729116/

49 Farmers and Hunters Feeding the Hungry (FHFH). Hunger in America. Webpage: https://www.fhfh.org/hunger-in-america.html?gclid=EAIaIQobChMIhLub2_-T6wIVodSzCh2TkgUpEAAYASAAEgKMJvD_BwE

50 Feeding America. Unemployment and poverty disproportionately affect African Americans — making combatting hunger even harder. Webpage: https://www.feedingamerica.org/hunger-in-america/african-american

51 doms-Young A, and Bruce MA. (2018). Examining the Impact of Structural Racism on Food Insecurity: Implications for Addressing Racial/Ethnic Disparities. *Family and Community Health* 41 Suppl(2 Suppl), Food Insecurity and Obesity (Suppl 2 FOOD INSECURITY AND OBESITY):S3-S6. Webpage: https://www.ncbi.nlm.nih.gov/pmc/articles/PMC5823283/

52 BrainyQuote.com. Michael Pollan Quotes. Webpage: https://www.brainyquote.com/quotes/michael_pollan_776580#:~:text=Michael%20

Pollan%20Quotes&text=Please%20enable%20Javascript-,We%20have%20
food%20deserts%20in%20our%20cities.,don't%20have%20grocery%20
stores.

[53] Kelli HM, Kim JH, Tahhan AS, et al. (2019). Living in Food Deserts and
Adverse Cardiovascular Outcomes in Patients With Cardiovascular Disease.
Journal of the American Heart Association (JAHA) 8(4) [open access]. Webpage:
https://www.ahajournals.org/doi/10.1161/JAHA.118.010694

[54] US Dept. of Health and Human Services (DHHS), Office of Minority Health.
Obesity and African Americans. Webpage: https://minorityhealth.hhs.gov/
omh/browse.aspx?lvl=4&lvlid=25

[55] Winkler MR, Bennett GG, and Brandon DH. (2017). Factors related to obesity and overweight among Black adolescent girls in the United States. *Women
and Health* 57(2): 208-248. Webpage: https://www.ncbi.nlm.nih.gov/pmc/
articles/PMC5050158/

[56] Yracheta JM, Lanaspa MA, MyPhuong, *et al.* (2015). Diabetes and
Kidney Disease in American Indians: Potential Role of Sugar-Sweetened
Beverages. *Mayo Clinic Proceedings* 90(6): 813-823. Webpage: https://
www.mayoclinicproceedings.org/article/S0025-6196(15)00268-2/pdf

[57] The March of Dimes. Low Birthweight. Webpage: https://
www.marchofdimes.org/complications/low-birthweight.aspx?gclid=EAIaI
QobChMIgOehrpKU6wIVuey1Ch3NVggVEAAYASAAEgJDv_D_BwE

[58] Centers for Disease Control (CDC). Folic Acid. Webpage: https://
www.cdc.gov/ncbddd/folicacid/about.html

[59] Commonwealth Fund. (November 20, 2018). Webpage: https://
www.commonwealthfund.org/blog/2018/public-charge-rule-negative-
impact-immigrants-health-care?gclid=EAIaIQobChMI0Py1x5aU6wIVL
AiICR2iZAWqEAAYASAAEgIUgfD_BwE

[60] Immigrant Legal Resource Center (ILRC). (August 19, 2020). Public Charge
Outreach Toolkit. Webpage: https://www.ilrc.org/public-charge-outreach-

toolkit?gclid=EAIaIQobChMI3cWI2JeU6wIVg56zCh2kdQLiEAAYBC
AAEgJ_AfD_BwE

61 Centers for Disease Control (CDC). U.S. Public Health Service Syphilis Study at Tuskegee. The Tuskegee Timeline. Webpage: https://www.cdc.gov/tuskegee/timeline.htm

62 Skloot, Rebecca. (2010). The Immortal Life of Henrietta Lacks. Crown Publishers: New York.

63 Stern AM. (2005). Sterilized in the name of public health: Race, immigration, and reproductive control in modern California. *American Journal of Public Health* 95(7): 1128-1138. Webpage: https://www.ncbi.nlm.nih.gov/pmc/articles/PMC1449330/

64 Krase K. (October 1, 2014). History of Forced Sterilization and Current U.S. Abuses. *Our Bodies, Ourselves* [Excerpt] Webpage: https://www.ourbodiesourselves.org/book-excerpts/health-article/forced-sterilization/

65 Southern Poverty Law Center. Landmark Case – Relf V. Weinberger. Webpage: https://www.splcenter.org/seeking-justice/case-docket/relf-v-weinberger

66 Kennedy EJ. (October 14, 2019). Community Voices – On Indigenous Peoples Day, recalling forced sterilizations of Native American women. MinnPost Webpage: https://www.minnpost.com/community-voices/2019/10/on-indigenous-peoples-day-recalling-forced-sterilizations-of-native-american-women/

67 National Public Radio (NPR). (March 7, 2016). The Supreme Court Ruling That Led To 70,000 Forced Sterilizations. Webpage: https://www.npr.org/sections/health-shots/2016/03/07/469478098/the-supreme-court-ruling-that-led-to-70-000-forced-sterilizations

68 Head T. (Updated November 23, 2018). Forced Sterilization in the United States. Webpage: https://www.thoughtco.com/forced-sterilization-in-united-states-721308

[69] Hoffman KM, Trawalter S, Axt JR, *et al.* (2016). Racial bias in pain assessment and treatment recommendations, and false beliefs about biological differences between blacks and whites. *Proceedings of the National Academy of Sciences of th USA* 113(16): 4296-4301. Webpage: https://www.ncbi.nlm.nih.gov/pmc/articles/PMC4843483/

[70] Association of American Medical Colleges (AAMC). (January 6, 2020). How we fail black patients in pain. Webpage: https://www.aamc.org/news-insights/how-we-fail-black-patients-pain

[71] Association of American Medical Colleges (AAMC). Diversity in Medicine: Facts and Figures 2019. Figure 18. Percentage of all active physicians by race/ethnicity, 2018. Webpage: https://www.aamc.org/data-reports/workforce/interactive-data/figure-18-percentage-all-active-physicians-race/ethnicity-2018

[72] Cuevas, Adolpho Gabriel [Portland State University, Portland, OR] (2013). Exploring Four Barriers Experienced by African Americans in Healthcare: Perceived Discrimination, Medical Mistrust, Race Discordance, and Poor Communication. [Dissertation] Webpage: https://pdxscholar.library.pdx.edu/cgi/viewcontent.cgi?article=1614&context=open_access_etds

[73] Hammond WP. (2010). Psychosocial correlates of medical mistrust among African American men. *American Journal of Community Psychology* 45(1-2): 87-106. Webpage: https://www.ncbi.nlm.nih.gov/pmc/articles/PMC2910212/

[74] Benjamin MR, and Middleton M. (April 25, 2019). Perceived discrimination in medical settings and perceived quality of care: A population-based study in Chicago. *PLoS One* [Open Access] Webpage: https://journals.plos.org/plosone/article?id=10.1371/journal.pone.0215976

[75] Benjamin MR, and Middleton M. (April 25, 2019). Perceived discrimination in medical settings and perceived quality of care: A population-based study

in Chicago. *PLoS One* [Open Access] Webpage: https://journals.plos.org/plosone/article?id=10.1371/journal.pone.0215976

76 Ross PT, Lypson ML, and Kumagi AK. (2012). Using illness narratives to explore African American perspectives of racial discrimination in healthcare. *Journal of Black Studies* 43(5): 520-544. Webpage: https://www.jstor.org/stable/23215232?seq=1

77 Serafini K, Coyer C, Brown Speights J, et al. (2020). Racism as Experienced by Physicians of Color in the Health Care Setting. *Family Medicine* 52(4): 282-287. Webpage: https://journals.stfm.org/familymedicine/2020/april/serafini-2019-0305/

78 Physicians News Network. (Updated January 31, 2017). New Survey Adds Race, Ethnicity to Questions of Physician Burnout. Webpage: http://www.physiciansnewsnetwork.com/la_county/new-survey-adds-race-ethnicity-to-questions-of-physician-burnout/article_eb1c00a2-e4bf-11e6-844f-fb6626a9fb63.html

79 Silver JK, Bean AC, Slocum C, *et al.* (July 15, 2019). Physician Workforce Disparities and Patient Care: A Narrative Review. Health Equity 3(1). [Open Access] Webpage: https://www.liebertpub.com/doi/full/10.1089/heq.2019.0040

80 AdvisoryBoard.com. (March 12, 2018). Racism still looms in hospital C-suites, Modern Healthcare reports. Webpage: https://www.advisory.com/daily-briefing/2018/03/12/c-suite-racism

81 Project Implicit [Harvard University]. Home Page. Webpage: https://implicit.harvard.edu/implicit/takeatest.html

82 Institute of Medicine (US) Committee on Understanding and Eliminating Racial and Ethnic Disparities in Health Care; Smedley BD, Stith AY, Nelson AR (Editors). (2003). Unequal Treatment: Confronting Racial and Ethnic Disparities in Health Care; Appendix D, Racial disparities in Health Care: Highlights From Focus Group Findings. Washington (DC): National

Academies Press (US). Webpage: https://www.ncbi.nlm.nih.gov/books/NBK220347/

[83] Smiley RA, Lauer P, Bienemy C, *et al.* (October 2018; updated 2019). The 2017 National Nursing Workforce Survey. *Journal of Nursing Regulation* 9(3-Supplement): S1-S88 Webpage: https://www.journalofnursingregulation.com/article/S2155-8256(18)30131-5/pdf

[84] MinorityNurse.com. Nursing Statistics. Webpage: https://minoritynurse.com/nursing-statistics/

[85] MinorityNurse.com. (April 15, 2019). Sexual Harassment by Patients: What Every Nurse Needs to Know. Webpage: https://minoritynurse.com/sexual-harassment-by-patients-what-every-nurse-needs-to-know/

[86] Centers for Disease Control (CDC). African Americans and Tobacco Use. Webpage: https://www.cdc.gov/tobacco/disparities/african-americans/index.htm

[87] TruthInitiative.org. (May 28, 2020). Tobacco use in the Hispanic/Latino American Community. Webpage: https://truthinitiative.org/research-resources/targeted-communities/tobacco-use-hispaniclatino-american-community

[88] American Lung Association. Tobacco Use in Racial and Ethnic Populations. Webpage: https://www.lung.org/quit-smoking/smoking-facts/impact-of-tobacco-use/tobacco-use-racial-and-ethnic

[89] TruthInitiative.org. (May 28, 2020). Tobacco use in the Hispanic/Latino American Community. Webpage: https://truthinitiative.org/research-resources/targeted-communities/tobacco-use-hispaniclatino-american-community

[90] Gopal SH, Mukherjee S, and Das SK. (2016). Direct and Second Hand Cigarette Smoke Exposure and Development of Childhood Asthma. *Journal of Environment and Health Science* 2(6):Direct and Second Hand Cigarette Smoke Exposure and Development of Childhood Asthma. Webpage: https://www.ncbi.nlm.nih.gov/pmc/articles/PMC5791751/

[91] Webb Hooper M, and Kolar SK. (2016). Racial/Ethnic Differences in Electronic Cigarette Use and Reasons for Use among Current and Former Smokers: Findings from a Community-Based Sample. *International Journal of Environmental Research and Public Health* 13(10): 1009. Webpage: https://www.ncbi.nlm.nih.gov/pmc/articles/PMC5086748/

[92] Webb Hooper M, and Kolar SK. (2016). Racial/Ethnic Differences in Electronic Cigarette Use and Reasons for Use among Current and Former Smokers: Findings from a Community-Based Sample. *International Journal of Environmental Research and Public Health* 13(10): 1009. Webpage: https://www.ncbi.nlm.nih.gov/pmc/articles/PMC5086748/

[93] Maron DF. (March 29, 2018). The Fight to Keep Tobacco Sacred. *Scientific American* Webpage: https://www.scientificamerican.com/article/the-fight-to-keep-tobacco-sacred/

[94] Cleveland Clinic (Cleveland, OH). Smoking. Webpage: https://my.clevelandclinic.org/health/articles/17488-smoking#:~:text=How%20smoking%20affects%20the%20heart,artery%20disease%20than%20do%20nonsmokers.

[95] Center for Disease Control (CDC). STATE System Medicaid Coverage of Tobacco Cessation Treatments Fact Sheet. Webpage: https://www.cdc.gov/statesystem/factsheets/medicaid/Cessation.html

[96] Hoffman J. (September 11, 2019). Purdue Pharma Tentatively Settles Thousands of Opioid Cases. *New York Times* Webpage: https://www.nytimes.com/2019/09/11/health/purdue-pharma-opioids-settlement.html

[97] Van Zee A. (2009). The promotion and marketing of oxycontin: commercial triumph, public health tragedy. *American Journal of Public Health*. 99(2): 221-227. Webpage: https://www.ncbi.nlm.nih.gov/pmc/articles/PMC2622774/

[98] Network of the National Library of Medicine, South Central Region [Blogadillo]. (February 8, 2018). Sickle Cell Anemia Predominant

Among African Americans. Webpage: https://news.nnlm.gov/scr/sickle-cell-anemia-predominant-among-african-americans/

[99] Johns Hopkins Medicine. (Fall 2016). Medical Rounds – Sickle Cell and Opioids. Webpage: https://www.hopkinsmedicine.org/news/publications/hopkins_medicine_magazine/medical_rounds/fall-2016/sickle-cell-and-opioids

[100] Balhara YPS, Singh S, and Kalra S. (February 2020). Pragmatic Opioid Use in Painful Diabetic Neuropathy.
European Endocrinology 16(1): 21-24. Webpage: https://www.touchendocrinology.com/diabetes/journal-articles/pragmatic-opioid-use-in-painful-diabetic-neuropathy/#article

[101] Somashekhar S. (April 4, 2016). The disturbing reason some African American patients may be undertreated for pain. *Washington Post* Webpage: https://www.washingtonpost.com/news/to-your-health/wp/2016/04/04/do-blacks-feel-less-pain-than-whites-their-doctors-may-think-so/

[102] Mosely T. (January 15, 2020). Black Americans Tend To Live With Unmanaged Pain When Under-Prescribed Opioids Due To Racial Bias, Experts Say. *WBUR* (Public Radio) Webpage: https://www.wbur.org/hereandnow/2020/01/15/black-americans-pain-opioids-racial-bias

[103] Cote E, Delaney TV, Hanna S, et al. (February 15, 2019). Vermont Dentists' Opinions and Attitudes Regarding the 2017 Opioid Prescribing Rules; Vermont Strategic Prevent Framework—Prescription Drugs (SPF-Rx) VDH Grant 03420-A18131S (UVM A.33338, P.034909): Report. [The University of Vermont, Larner College of Medicine, Burlington, VT]. Webpage: https://www.healthvermont.gov/sites/default/files/documents/pdf/ADAP_Dental_Opioid_Rx_Rule_Survey_Report_2019_02_19.pdf

[104] National Council for Behavioral Health. Stigma Regarding Mental Illness among People of Color. Webpage:

https://www.thenationalcouncil.org/BH365/2019/07/08/ stigma-regarding-mental-illness-among-people-of-color/

[105] National Institute of Mental Health (NIMH). Major Depression. Webpage: https://www.nimh.nih.gov/health/statistics/major-depression.shtml

[106] MentalHealthAmerica. Black And African American Communities And Mental Health. Webpage: https://www.mhanational.org/issues/ black-and-african-american-communities-and-mental-health

[107] National Alliance on Mental Illness (NAMI). Black/African American. Webpage: https://www.nami.org/Your-Journey/ Identity-and-Cultural-Dimensions/Black-African-American

[108] Anxiety and Depression Association of America. Latinx/Hispanic Communities. Webpage: https://adaa.org/finding-help/hispanic-latinos

[109] US DHHS, Office of Minority Health. Mental and Behavioral Health – African Americans. Webpage: https://minorityhealth.hhs.gov/omh/ browse.aspx?lvl=4&lvlid=24

[110] University of Michigan, Institute for Healthcare Policy and Innovation. (September 16, 2016). Black Americans may be more resilient to stress than white Americans. Webpage: https://ihpi.umich.edu/news/ black-americans-may-be-more-resilient-stress-white-americans

[111] Centers for Disease Control (CDC). National Center for Health Statistics. (June 2015). Data Brief – Racial and Ethnic Disparities in Men's Use of Mental Health Treatments. Webpage: https://www.cdc.gov/nchs/products/ databriefs/db206.htm

[112] US Dept. of Health and Human Services (DHHS). Mental Health and Substance Abuse – Does depression increase the risk for suicide? Webpage: https://www.hhs.gov/answers/mental-health-and-substance-abuse/does-depression-increase-risk-of-suicide/index.html

[113] Sohail Z, Bailey RK, and Richie WD. (2014). Misconceptions of depression in African Americans. *Frontiers in Psychiatry* 5: 65. Webpage: https://www.ncbi.nlm.nih.gov/pmc/articles/PMC4064454/

[114] Himle JA, Baser RE, Taylor RJ, *et al.* (2009). Anxiety disorders among African Americans, blacks of Caribbean descent, and non-Hispanic whites in the United States. *Journal of Anxiety Disorders* 23(5): 578-590. Webpage: https://www.ncbi.nlm.nih.gov/pmc/articles/PMC4187248/

[115] Smith JP, Randall CL. (2012). Anxiety and alcohol use disorders: comorbidity and treatment considerations. *Alcohol Research: Current Reviews* 34(4): 414-431. Webpage: https://www.ncbi.nlm.nih.gov/pmc/articles/PMC3860396/

[116] Anxiety and Depression Association of America. Understanding the Facts. Understanding the Facts of Anxiety Disorders and Depression is the First Step. Webpage: https://adaa.org/understanding-anxiety?gclid=EAIaIQobChMIqPbFzreb6wIVOQiICR2-pwyDEAAYASAAEgJOifD_BwE

[117] Celestine S. (December 4, 2019). African Americans Face Unique Mental Health Risks. *WebMed.com* Webpage: https://www.webmd.com/mental-health/news/20191204/african-americans-face-unique-mental-health-risks

[118] Akinhanmi MO, Biernacka JM, Strakowski SM, et al. (2018). Racial disparities in bipolar disorder treatment and research: a call to action. *Bipolar Disorders*. 20(6): 506-514. Webpage: https://www.ncbi.nlm.nih.gov/pmc/articles/PMC6175457/

[119] American Psychiatric Association. What is Schizophrenia? Webpage: https://www.psychiatry.org/patients-families/schizophrenia/what-is-schizophrenia

[120] Horvitz-Lennon M, McGuire TG, Alegria M, *et al.* (2009). Racial and ethnic disparities in the treatment of a Medicaid population with schizophrenia. *Health Services Research* 44(6): 2106-2122. Webpage: https://www.ncbi.nlm.nih.gov/pmc/articles/PMC2796317/

[121] Human Rights (October 21, 2003). Watch. Ill-equipped: U.S. pris-

ons and offenders with mental illness. Webpage: https://www.hrw.org/report/2003/10/21/ill-equipped/us-prisons-and-offenders-mental-illness

[122] Oluwoye O, Stiles B, Monroe-DeVita M, *et al.* (2018). Racial-Ethnic Disparities in First-Episode Psychosis Treatment Outcomes From the RAISE-ETP Study. Psychiatric Services 69(11): 1138-1145. Webpage: https://ps.psychiatryonline.org/doi/pdf/10.1176/appi.ps.201800067

[123] Cook BL, and Alegría M. (2011). Racial-ethnic disparities in substance abuse treatment: The role of criminal history and socioeconomic status. *Psychiatric Services (Washington DC)* 62(11): 1273-1281. Webpage: https://www.ncbi.nlm.nih.gov/pmc/articles/PMC3665009/

[124] Los Angeles Times. (January 2, 1990). Drug Plague a Racist Conspiracy? Crack: Some blacks suspect that the white Establishment encourages or at least tolerates the epidemic of drugs and violence in black communities. Webpage: https://www.latimes.com/archives/la-xpm-1990-01-02-vw-195-story.html

[125] US DHHS, Substance Abuse and Mental Health Services Administration (SAMHSA). 2018 National Survey on Drug Use and Health (NSDUH): African Americans. Webpage: https://www.samhsa.gov/data/sites/default/files/reports/rpt23247/2_AfricanAmerican_2020_01_14_508.pdf

[126] US DHHS, Substance Abuse and Mental Health Services Administration (SAMHSA). 2018 National Survey on Drug Use and Health (NSDUH): Hispanics, Latino or Spanish Origin or Descent. Webpage: https://www.samhsa.gov/data/sites/default/files/reports/rpt23249/4_Hispanic_2020_01_14_508.pdf

[127] Center on Budget and Policy Priorities (CBPP). Trump Administration's Harmful Changes to Medicaid. Webpage: https://www.cbpp.org/research/health/trump-administrations-harmful-changes-to-medicaid

[128] US Agency for Healthcare Research and Quality (AHRQ). 2017 National

Healthcare Quality and Disparities Report. Webpage: https://www.ahrq.gov/research/findings/nhqrdr/nhqdr17/index.html

[129] US Department of Veterans Affairs. (March, 2017). Minority Veterans Report: Military Service History and VA Benefit Utilization Statistics. Webpage: https://www.va.gov/vetdata/docs/SpecialReports/Minority_Veterans_Report.pdf

[130] Duke Clinical Research Institute. Depression linked to worse outcomes in African Americans with heart failure. Webpage: https://dcri.org/depression-linked-worse-outcomes-african-americans-heart-failure/

[131] Allen SA, Wakeman SE, Cohen RL, *et al.* (2010). Physicians in US Prisons in the Era of Mass Incarceration. *International Journal of Prisoner Health* 6(3): 100-106. Webpage: https://www.ncbi.nlm.nih.gov/pmc/articles/PMC3204660/

[132] The Sentencing Project. (June 14, 2016). The Color of Justice: Racial and Ethnic Disparity in State Prisons. Webpage: https://www.sentencingproject.org/publications/color-of-justice-racial-and-ethnic-disparity-in-state-prisons/

[133] The Sentencing Project. (June 14, 2016). The Color of Justice: Racial and Ethnic Disparity in State Prisons. Webpage: https://www.sentencingproject.org/publications/color-of-justice-racial-and-ethnic-disparity-in-state-prisons/

[134] University of California, Berkeley (Berkeley Political Review). (January 28, 2017). Convicts without Care: How the Privatization of Healthcare in the U.S. Prison System Fails to Protect Inmates' Health. Webpage: https://bpr.berkeley.edu/2017/01/28/convicts-without-care-how-the-privatization-of-healthcare-in-the-u-s-prison-system-fails-to-protect-inmates-health/

[135] University of California, Berkeley (Berkeley Political Review). (January 28, 2017). Convicts without Care: How the Privatization of Healthcare in the U.S. Prison System Fails to Protect Inmates' Health. Webpage: https://bpr.berkeley.edu/2017/01/28/convicts-without-care-how-the-privatization-of-healthcare-in-the-u-s-prison-system-fails-to-protect-inmates-health/

136 Linder M. (February 11, 2018). Opinion; Scholastic Award Winners. "Mass Incarceration Nation: The Truth Behind Reagan's War on Drugs". *Bancroft School* Webpage: https://unleashed.bancroftschool.org/3562/opinion/mass-incarceration-nation-the-truth-behind-reagans-war-on-drugs/

137 Allen SA, Wakeman SE, Cohen RL, *et al.* (2010). Physicians in US Prisons in the Era of Mass Incarceration. *International Journal of Prisoner Health* 6(3): 100-106. Webpage: https://www.ncbi.nlm.nih.gov/pmc/articles/PMC3204660/

138 Valera P, Chang Y, and Lian Z. (2017). HIV risk inside U.S. prisons: A systematic review of risk reduction interventions conducted in U.S. prisons. *AIDS Care* 29(8): 943-952. Webpage: https://www.ncbi.nlm.nih.gov/pmc/articles/PMC5587216/

139 Lambert LA, Armstrong LR, Lobato MN, *et al.* (2016). Tuberculosis in Jails and Prisons: United States, 2002-2013. *American Journal of Public Health* 106(12): 2231-2237. Webpage: https://www.ncbi.nlm.nih.gov/pmc/articles/PMC5104991/

140 Centers for Disease Control (CDC). TB in Correctional Facilities in the United States. Webpage: https://www.cdc.gov/tb/topic/populations/correctional/default.htm

141 Hausman S. (January 9, 2014). 30,000 Inmates, 40 Doctors: Health Care Remains A Concern At Virginia Prisons. *WAMU 88.5 - American Friend Radio.* Webpage: https://wamu.org/story/14/01/09/30000_inmates_40_doctors_health_care_remains_a_concern_at_virginia_prisons/

142 Almost J, Gifford WA, Doran D, *et al.* (2013). Correctional nursing: A study protocol to develop an educational intervention to optimize nursing practice in a unique context. *Implementation Science*;8: 71. Webpage: https://www.ncbi.nlm.nih.gov/pmc/articles/PMC3691633/

143 Population Reference Bureau. Parents' Imprisonment Linked to Children's Health, Behavioral Problems. Webpage: https://www.prb.org/incarcerated-

parents-and-childrens-health/#:~:text=In%20particular%2C%20 children%20with%20an,ADD%2FADHD%2C%20and%20anxiety.

[144] Bekiempis V. (July 22, 2015). Don't Get Cancer if You're in Prison. *Newsweek* Webpage: https://www.newsweek.com/2015/07/31/dont-get-cancer-if-youre-prison-356010.html

[145] Fitzgerald K. (November 20, 2019). Women in Prison Have Increased Rates of HPV, Cervical Cancer. *DocWireNews.com* Webpage: https://www.docwirenews.com/docwire-pick/hem-onc-picks/women-in-prison-have-increased-rates-of-hpv-cervical-cancer/#:~:text=Women%20in%20 Prison%20Have%20Increased%20Rates%20of%20HPV%2C%20 Cervical%20Cancer,-By&text=Imprisoned%20women%20are%20at%20 higher,Journal%20of%20Epidemiology%20%26%20Community%20 Health.

[146] Brookings Institute. (May 15, 2020). Webinar: The impact of COVID-19 on prisons. Webpage: https://www.brookings.edu/events/ the-impact-of-covid-19-on-prisons/

[147] National Public Radio (NPR). (June 15, 2020). https:// www.npr.org/2020/06/15/877457603/as-covid-spreads-in-u-s-prisons-lockdowns-spark-fear-of-more-solitary-confinemen

[148] National Public Radio (NPR). (May 16, 2016). Despite $10B 'Fix,' Veterans Are Waiting Even Longer To See Doctors. Webpage: https://www.npr.org/sections/health-shots/2016/05/16/477814218/ attempted-fix-for-va-health-delays-creates-new-bureaucracy

[149] American Public Health Association. (November 18, 2014). Removing Barriers to Mental Health Services for Veterans. Webpage: https:// www.apha.org/policies-and-advocacy/public-health-policy-statements/ policy-database/2015/01/28/14/51/removing-barriers-to-mental-health-services-for-veterans#:~:text=Veterans%20have%20disproportionate%20 rates%20of,anxiety%2C%20and%20military%20sexual%20trauma.

150 American Public Health Association. (November 18, 2014). Removing Barriers to Mental Health Services for Veterans. Webpage: https://www.apha.org/policies-and-advocacy/public-health-policy-statements/policy-database/2015/01/28/14/51/removing-barriers-to-mental-health-services-for-veterans#:~:text=Veterans%20have%20disproportionate%20rates%20of,anxiety%2C%20and%20military%20sexual%20trauma.

151 US Dept. of Veterans Affairs, Office of Mental Health and Suicide Prevention. 2019 National Suicide Prevention Annual Report. Webpage: https://www.mentalhealth.va.gov/docs/data-sheets/2019/2019_National_Veteran_Suicide_Prevention_Annual_Report_508.pdf

152 US Dept. of Veterans Affairs, Office of Mental Health and Suicide Prevention. 2019 National Suicide Prevention Annual Report. Webpage: https://www.mentalhealth.va.gov/docs/data-sheets/2019/2019_National_Veteran_Suicide_Prevention_Annual_Report_508.pdf

153 Hester RD. (2017). Lack of access to mental health services contributing to the high suicide rates among veterans. *International Journal of Mental Health Systems* 11: 47. Webpage: https://www.ncbi.nlm.nih.gov/pmc/articles/PMC5563010/

154 US Dept. of Veterans Affairs (VA). (March 2017). Minority Veterans Report: Military Service History and VA Benefit Utilization Statistics. Webpage: https://www.va.gov/vetdata/docs/SpecialReports/Minority_Veterans_Report.pdf

155 Steinhauer J. (January 30, 2019). Veterans Will Have More Access to Private Health Care Under New V.A. Rules. *New York Times* Webpage: https://www.nytimes.com/2019/01/30/us/politics/veterans-health-care.html

156 Rand Corporation. (2019). Research Brief – Improving the Quality of Mental Health Care for Veterans: Lessons from RAND Research. Santa Monica, CA: Rand Corporation. Webpage: https://www.rand.org/pubs/research_briefs/RB10087.html

[157] National Foundation for Transplants. Get Informed. Webpage: https://transplants.org/get-informed/?gclid=EAIaIQobChMI4P_Pjomo6wIVA4bICh2AiwEGEAAYASAAEgKof_D_BwE

[158] Debt.org. Hospital and Surgery Costs. Webpage: https://www.debt.org/medical/hospital-surgery-costs/#:~:text=Hospital%20costs%20averaged%20%243%2C949%20per,are%20related%20to%20medical%20expenses.

[159] Castillo M. (January 2, 2014). Cost of an appendectomy? Reddit user posts $55,000 bill. *CBS News* Webpage: https://www.cbsnews.com/news/cost-of-an-appendectomy-reddit-user-posts-55000-bill/

[160] Debt.org. Hospital and Surgery Costs. Webpage: https://www.debt.org/medical/hospital-surgery-costs/#:~:text=Hospital%20costs%20averaged%20%243%2C949%20per,are%20related%20to%20medical%20expenses.

[161] Kaiser Family Foundation (KFF). The Uninsured and the ACA: A Primer - Key Facts about Health Insurance and the Uninsured amidst Changes to the Affordable Care Act. Webpage: https://www.kff.org/report-section/the-uninsured-and-the-aca-a-primer-key-facts-about-health-insurance-and-the-uninsured-amidst-changes-to-the-affordable-care-act-what-are-the-financial-implications-of-lacking-insu/

[162] Kaiser Family Foundation (KFF). The Uninsured and the ACA: A Primer - Key Facts about Health Insurance and the Uninsured amidst Changes to the Affordable Care Act. Webpage: https://www.kff.org/report-section/the-uninsured-and-the-aca-a-primer-key-facts-about-health-insurance-and-the-uninsured-amidst-changes-to-the-affordable-care-act-what-are-the-financial-implications-of-lacking-insu/

[163] Center on Budget and Policy Priorities. (March 19, 2019). Chart Book: Accomplishments of Affordable Care Act. Webpage: https://www.cbpp.org/research/health/chart-book-accomplishments-of-affordable-care-act

[164] Kaiser Family Foundation (KFF). Medicaid – The Coverage Gap: Uninsured Poor Adults in States that Do Not Expand Medicaid. Webpage: https://

www.kff.org/medicaid/issue-brief/the-coverage-gap-uninsured-poor-adults-in-states-that-do-not-expand-medicaid/

[165] Center on Budget and Policy Priorities. (March 19, 2019). Chart Book: Accomplishments of Affordable Care Act. Webpage: https://www.cbpp.org/research/health/chart-book-accomplishments-of-affordable-care-act

[166] Brookings Institute. (February 19, 2020). There are clear, race-based inequalities in health insurance and health outcomes. Webpage: https://www.brookings.edu/blog/usc-brookings-schaeffer-on-health-policy/2020/02/19/there-are-clear-race-based-inequalities-in-health-insurance-and-health-outcomes/

[167] US Census Bureau. (September 12, 2018). Health Insurance Coverage in the United States: 2017. Webpage: https://www.census.gov/library/publications/2018/demo/p60-264.html

[168] Kaiser Family Foundation (KFF). Medicaid – The Coverage Gap: Uninsured Poor Adults in States that Do Not Expand Medicaid. Webpage: https://www.kff.org/medicaid/issue-brief/the-coverage-gap-uninsured-poor-adults-in-states-that-do-not-expand-medicaid/

[169] Kaiser Family Foundation (KFF). Medicaid – The Coverage Gap: Uninsured Poor Adults in States that Do Not Expand Medicaid. Webpage: https://www.kff.org/medicaid/issue-brief/the-coverage-gap-uninsured-poor-adults-in-states-that-do-not-expand-medicaid/

[170] Pear R. (November 29, 2016). Tom Price, H.H.S. Nominee, Drafted Remake of Health Law. *New York Times* Webpage: https://www.nytimes.com/2016/11/29/us/tom-price-trump-health-secretary.html

[171] FreshBooks.com. Do Small Businesses Have to Offer Health Insurance? A Guide to Employee Health Benefits. Webpage: https://www.freshbooks.com/hub/insurance/do-small-businesses-have-to-offer-health-insurance

[172] Centers for Medicare and Medicaid Services (CMS), Center for Consumer Information and Insurance Oversight. The Mental Health Parity and Addic-

tion Equity Act (MHPAEA). Webpage: https://www.cms.gov/CCIIO/
Programs-and-Initiatives/Other-Insurance-Protections/mhpaea_factsheet

[173] Association of Health Care Journalists (AHCJ). (January 21, 2020). Report
shows health insurers are failing to comply with mental health parity laws.
Webpage: https://healthjournalism.org/blog/2020/01/report-shows-health-
insurers-are-failing-to-comply-with-mental-health-parity-laws/

[174] Melek S, Davenport S, and Gray TJ. (November 19, 2019). Milliman
Research Report – Addiction and mental health vs. physical health: Widening
disparities in network use and provider reimbursement. *Milliman* Webpage:
http://assets.milliman.com/ektron/Addiction_and_mental_health_vs_
physical_health_Widening_disparities_in_network_use_and_provider_
reimbursement.pdf

[175] Oprah.com. Why Finding a Therapist Can Be Especially Hard for
Black Women. Webpage: http://www.oprah.com/health_wellness/
how-racial-bias-affects-mental-health-treatment

[176] American Psychological Association (APA). (June 2018). Spanish-speaking
psychologists in demand. *Monitor on Psychology* 49(6): 68. Webpage: https://
www.apa.org/monitor/2018/06/spanish-speaking#:~:text=A%20rare%20
commodity&text=Yet%20there%20are%20only%20about,ago%2C%20
according%20to%20Census%20data.

[177] Medicaid and CHIP Payment and Access Commission (MACPAC).
(December 2018). MACSTats: Medicaid and CHIP Data Book. Webpage:
https://www.macpac.gov/wp-content/uploads/2018/12/December-2018-
MACStats-Data-Book.pdf

[178] National Committee to Preserve Social Security and Medicare. African
Americans and Medicare. Webpage: https://www.ncpssm.org/documents/
medicare-policy-papers/medicare-medicaid-important-african-americans/

[179] Medicaid and CHIP Payment and Access Commission (MACPAC).
(December 2018). MACSTats: Medicaid and CHIP Data Book. Webpage:

https://www.macpac.gov/wp-content/uploads/2018/12/December-2018-MACStats-Data-Book.pdf

[180] Center on Budget and Policy Priorities. Medicaid Works for People with Disabilities. Webpage: https://www.cbpp.org/research/health/medicaid-works-for-people-with-disabilities

[181] Medicaid and CHIP Payment and Access Commission (MACPAC). (December 2018). MACSTats: Medicaid and CHIP Data Book. Webpage: https://www.macpac.gov/wp-content/uploads/2018/12/December-2018-MACStats-Data-Book.pdf

[182] Gordon SH, Gadbois EA, Shield RR, *et al.* (2018). Qualitative perspectives of primary care providers who treat Medicaid managed care patients. *BMC Health Services Research* 18(1): 728. Webpage: https://www.ncbi.nlm.nih.gov/pmc/articles/PMC6150984/

[183] Medicaid and CHIP Payment and Access Commission (MACPAC). (December 2018). MACSTats: Medicaid and CHIP Data Book. Webpage: https://www.macpac.gov/wp-content/uploads/2018/12/December-2018-MACStats-Data-Book.pdf

[184] Niess MA, Blair IV, Furniss A, et al. (2018). Specialty Physician Attitudes and Beliefs about Medicaid Patients. *Journal of Family Medicine* 5(3). (Open Access) Webpage: https://austinpublishinggroup.com/family-medicine/fulltext/jfm-v5-id1141.php

[185] Medicaid and CHIP Payment and Access Commission (MACPAC). (December 2018). MACSTats: Medicaid and CHIP Data Book. Webpage: https://www.macpac.gov/wp-content/uploads/2018/12/December-2018-MACStats-Data-Book.pdf

[186] Kaiser Family Foundation (KFF). 10 Things to Know about Medicaid: Setting the Facts Straight. Webpage: https://www.kff.org/medicaid/issue-brief/10-things-to-know-about-medicaid-setting-the-facts-straight/?gclid

=EAIaIQobChMIsoDY7bGo6wIVBO21Ch1ueQYkEAAYASAAEgLm
ffD_BwE

[187] Niess MA, Blair IV, Furniss A, et al. (2018). Specialty Physician Attitudes and Beliefs about Medicaid Patients. *Journal of Family Medicine* 5(3). (Open Access) Webpage: https://austinpublishinggroup.com/family-medicine/fulltext/jfm-v5-id1141.php

[188] US Dept. of Health and Human Services, HRSA Health Center Program. What is a Health Center? Webpage: https://bphc.hrsa.gov/about/what-is-a-health-center/index.html

[189] National Association of Community Health Centers. Medicaid and Medicare. Webpage: http://www.nachc.org/focus-areas/policy-matters/medicaid-and-medicare/

[190] American Public Health Association (APHA). (May 2019). President's budget would hinder US public health progress: Huge cuts proposed. *The Nations Health* 49(3): 1-14. Webpage: https://thenationshealth.aphapublications.org/content/49/3/1.2

[191] Pew Charitable Trusts. (May 9, 2018). Work Requirements for Medicaid Are Now OK in Four States. Webpage: https://www.pewtrusts.org/en/research-and-analysis/blogs/stateline/2018/05/09/work-requirements-for-medicaid-are-now-ok-in-four-states

[192] National Public Radio (NPR). (February 14, 2020). U.S. Appeals Court Upholds Ruling Blocking States' Medicaid Work Requirements. Webpage: https://www.npr.org/sections/health-shots/2020/02/14/806119263/federal-appeals-court-upholds-ruling-blocking-medicaid-work-requirements

[193] National Public Radio (NPR). (February 18, 2019). In Arkansas, Thousands Of People Have Lost Medicaid Coverage Over New Work Rule. Webpage: https://www.npr.org/sections/health-shots/2019/02/18/694504586/in-arkansas-thousands-of-people-have-lost-medicaid-coverage-over-new-work-rule

[194] Milbank Memorial Fund. (September 2018). Surprising Statistics on the Uninsured. *The Milbank Quarterly* 96 Webpage: https://www.milbank.org/quarterly/articles/surprising-statistics-on-the-uninsured/?gclid=EAIaIQob ChMI1Z6K-N6o6wIVcQiICR27LgvmEAAYASAAEgJfzfD_BwE

[195] Kaiser Family Foundation. (December 13, 2019). Key Facts about the Uninsured Population. Webpage: https://www.kff.org/uninsured/issue-brief/key-facts-about-the-uninsured-population/

[196] Kaiser Family Foundation. (December 13, 2019). Key Facts about the Uninsured Population. Webpage: https://www.kff.org/uninsured/issue-brief/key-facts-about-the-uninsured-population/

[197] Kaiser Familiy Foundation (KFF). (March 18, 2020). Health Coverage of Immigrants. Webpage: https://www.kff.org/disparities-policy/fact-sheet/health-coverage-of-immigrants/

[198] HealthcareDive.com. Fewer uninsured ED visits, hospitalizations after ACA, JAMA study finds. Webpage: https://www.healthcaredive.com/news/fewer-uninsured-ed-visits-hospitalizations-after-aca-jama-study-finds/553075/

[199] Society for Human Resource Management (SHRM). (June 30, 2020). Sparring over ACA Picks Up Before 2021 Supreme Court Ruling. Webpage: https://www.shrm.org/resourcesandtools/hr-topics/benefits/pages/sparring-over-aca-picks-up-before-2021-supreme-court-ruling.aspx

[200] Baker M, and Fink S. (April 22, 2020). Covid 19 Arrived in Seattle. Where It Went From There Stunned Scientists. New York Times Webpage: https://www.nytimes.com/2020/04/22/us/coronavirus-sequencing.html

[201] Dyal NP. (March 3, 2020). First Case of COVID-19 in NYC, First Death Reported in Washington State. *InfectiousDiseaseAdvisor.com* Webpage: https://www.infectiousdiseaseadvisor.com/home/topics/respiratory/first-case-of-covid-19-in-nyc-first-death-reported-in-washington-state/

[202] Human Rights Watch (HRW). (May 12, 2020). Covid-

19 Fueling Anti-Asian Racism and Xenophobia World-wide. Webpage: https://www.hrw.org/news/2020/05/12/covid-19-fueling-anti-asian-racism-and-xenophobia-worldwide

203 World Health Organization (WHO). International Travel and Health. SARS (Severe Acute Respiratory Syndrome). Webpage: https://www.who.int/ith/diseases/sars/en/

204 Bean M. (March 12, 2020). A look back at swine flu: 8 facts about the world's last pandemic in 2009. *Becker's Hospital Review* Webpage: https://www.beckershospitalreview.com/public-health/swine-flu-8-facts-about-the-world-s-last-pandemic-in-2009.html

205 World Health Organization (WHO). Middle East respiratory syndrome coronavirus (MERS-CoV). Webpage: https://www.who.int/emergencies/mers-cov/en/

206 Petrosillo N, Viceconte G, Ergonul O, *et al.* (2020). COVID-19, SARS and MERS: Are they closely related?. *Clinical Microbiology and Infection* 26(6): 729-734. Webpage: https://www.ncbi.nlm.nih.gov/pmc/articles/PMC7176926/

207 Centers for Disease Control (CDC). What is Ebola Virus Disease? Webpage: https://www.cdc.gov/vhf/ebola/about.html

208 World Health Organization. Newsroom – 10th Ebola outbreak in the Democratic Republic of the Congo declared over; vigilance against flare-ups and support for survivors must continue. Webpage: https://www.who.int/news-room/detail/25-06-2020-10th-ebola-outbreak-in-the-democratic-republic-of-the-congo-declared-over-vigilance-against-flare-ups-and-support-for-survivors--must-continue

209 Centers for Disease Control (CDC). COVID-19 Hospitalization and Death by Race/Ethnicity. Webpage: https://www.cdc.gov/coronavirus/2019-ncov/covid-data/investigations-discovery/hospitalization-death-by-race-ethnicity.html

210 Centers for Disease Control (CDC). COVID-19 Hospitalization and Death by Race/Ethnicity. Webpage: https://www.cdc.gov/coronavirus/2019-ncov/covid-data/investigations-discovery/hospitalization-death-by-race-ethnicity.html

211 The Commonwealth Fund. (April 23, 2020). To the Point – Quick Takes on Health Care Policy and Practice. COVID-19 More Prevalent, Deadlier in U.S. Counties with Higher Black Populations. Webpage: https://www.commonwealthfund.org/blog/2020/covid-19-more-prevalent-deadlier-us-counties-higher-black-populations?gclid=EAIaIQobChMIj522o72q6wIVD7bICh28lgetEAAYASAAEgI_tPD_BwE

212 APM Research Lab. The Color of Coronavirus: COVID-19 Deaths by Race and Ethnicity in the U.S. Webpage: https://www.apmresearchlab.org/covid/deaths-by-race#black

213 Marguerite Casey Foundation. (April 22, 2020). Marguerite Casey Foundation Announces $3.5 Million in COVID-19 Grant. Webpage: https://caseygrants.org/who-we-are/inside-mcf/marguerite-casey-foundation-announces-3-5-million-in-covid-19-grant-funding-to-tackle-racial-disparities-resulting-from-pandemic/?gclid=EAIaIQobChMI7P_6iL2q6wIVE26GCh1fJAFeEAAYASAAEgJLsPD_BwE

214 Mayo Clinic. Coronavirus infection by race: What's behind the health disparities? Webpage: https://www.mayoclinic.org/diseases-conditions/coronavirus/expert-answers/coronavirus-infection-by-race/faq-20488802

215 CNBC News. (July 17, 2020). The $600 unemployment payments are likely ending. Here's why. Webpage: https://www.cnbc.com/2020/07/17/why-republicans-dont-want-to-extend-the-600-unemployment-payments.html

216 Proctor D. (February 10, 2015). Culture of Health Blog — A New Approach to Eliminating Health Disparities. *Robert Wood Johnson Foundation* Webpage: https://www.rwjf.org/en/blog/2015/02/let_s_eliminate_heal.html

[217] National Center for Complementary and Integrative Health. Meditation: In-Depth. Webpage: https://www.nccih.nih.gov/health/meditation-in-depth

[218] American Medical Association (AMA). (May 22, 2018). Navigating state medical licensure. Webpage: https://www.ama-assn.org/residents-students/career-planning-resource/navigating-state-medical-licensure

[219] Medicare.gov. Physician Compare. Find Medicare physicians & other clinicians. Webpage: https://www.medicare.gov/physiciancompare/

[220] Jacobs B, Ryan AM, Henrichs KS, *et al.* (2018). Medical Interpreters in Outpatient Practice. *Annals of Family Medicine* 16(1): 70-76. Webpage: https://www.ncbi.nlm.nih.gov/pmc/articles/PMC5758324/

[221] New York Magazine. (June 5, 2020). 7 Anti-Racist Books Recommended by Educators and Activists. *The Strategist* Webpage: https://nymag.com/strategist/article/anti-racist-reading-list.html

[222] Massari, Allison. Compassion as a Healing Tool. Webpage: https://allisonmassari.com/compassion-as-a-healing-tool

[223] Love B, and Hayes-Greene D [Racial Equity Institute]. The Groundwater Approach: Building a Practical Understanding of Structural Racism. Webpage: https://www.racialequityinstitute.com/groundwaterapproach

[224] Love B, and Hayes-Greene D [Racial Equity Institute]. The Groundwater Approach: Building a Practical Understanding of Structural Racism. *(Page 5)* Webpage: https://www.racialequityinstitute.com/groundwaterapproach

[225] Andrews PE. (Spring, 2004). Reparations for Apartheids Victims: The Path to Reconciliation? *DePaul Law Review* 53(3): 1155. Webpage: https://via.library.depaul.edu/cgi/viewcontent.cgi?article=1465&context=law-review

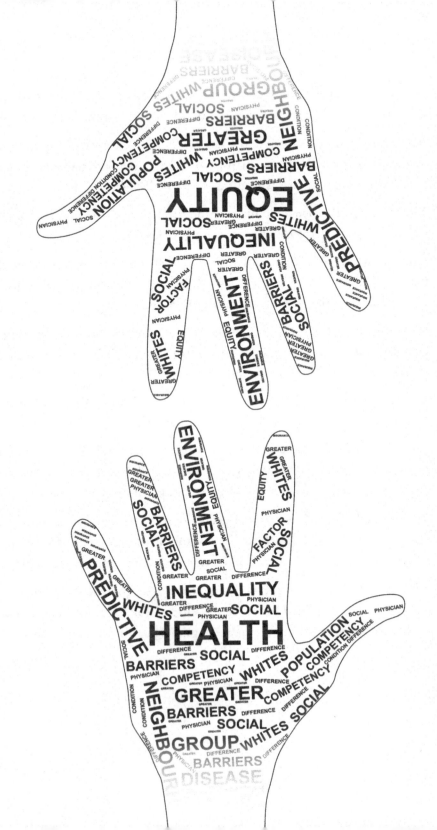